Psychodrama

PSYCHODRAMA

Resolving Emotional Problems Through Role-Playing

LEWIS YABLONSKY

BRUNNER/MAZEL *Publishers* • New York

First Brunner/Mazel Edition 1992

Library of Congress Cataloging in Publication Data

Yablonsky, Lewis
  Psychodrama: resolving emotional problems
through role-playing
  Includes index.
    1. Psychodrama. I. Title. [DNLM: 1. Role-playing —
Popular works. 2. Mental disorders — Therapy — Popular
works. WM430   Y11p]
  RC489.P7Y3   616.8'915   75-36385

ISBN: 0-87630-698-9

Published by
BRUNNER/MAZEL, INC.
19 Union Square West
New York, New York 10003

Manufactured in the United States of America

10 9 8 7 6 5 4 3 2 1

CONTENTS

Contents

CHAPTER 7

EPILOGUE

ACKNOWLEDGMENTS

SINCE 1949 I have directed or participated in several thousand psychodrama sessions. All of the participants in all of these sessions have contributed to this book.

I was fortunate during this twenty-five year period to be first a student and later a colleague of the founder and master of psychodrama, J. L. Moreno, M.D. (1889–1974). This book is gratefully dedicated to J. L. and Zerka Moreno, whose teachings and spirit continue to infuse the worldwide psychodrama and group psychotherapy movement.

My wife, Donna, has been my psychodrama partner and best friend since we met—in a psychodrama session, of course—back in 1961. Her remarkable perceptions as a psychodramatist are incorporated into many concepts in this work. In particular, she wrote several poignant vignettes, which are part of the chapter on psychodramatic scenarios.

My son, Mitch, now twelve, has role-trained me as effectively as he could on how to parent, and his beautiful spirit and presence have helped me immensely in the practice of psychodrama. As a result of many sessions, I have learned to appreciate my wonderful parents, who in their own way helped to develop my awareness of group process.

My editor, Farrell Wallerstein, has helped me to sharpen the book in many ways—especially through her creative suggestion to add the chapter on relating psychodrama to other therapeutic modalities. In all cases where I have used actual case histories, I have changed names and, to some degree, the circumstances of the session so that no one's identity can be recognized.

I am immensely grateful to all of the loving people who made this book possible.

Lewis Yablonsky, Ph.D.
California State University
Northridge, California

Psychodrama

CHAPTER

1

Participating in Psychodrama

PSYCHODRAMA is a natural and automatic process. Everyone at some time has an inner drama going on in his mind. In this confidential setting you are the star of your psychodrama session and play all of the roles. The others you encounter in your monodrama may be your parents, an employer, a God you love or one who has forsaken you, a wife, husband, or lover who has rejected you or demands more than you are willing to give. The others, or, as they are called in psychodrama, your auxiliary egos, may not be actual human adversaries but some ideal someone or something you want but cannot have—an unfulfilled dream, or perhaps an obsession for fame or wealth.

Many people are able to act out these internal psychodramas in the reality and activity of their external life. For such people, psychodrama is not a necessary vehicle except as an interesting adjunct to their life experiences. But for most people, psychodrama can provide a unique opportunity for *externalizing* their internal world onto a theatrical stage of life; and, with the help of the group present at a session, emotional conflicts and problems can often be resolved.

A basic theme of this book is that of psychodrama as a happening or as a productive *experience* rather than exclusively as a therapeutic method, even though a significant side effect of psychodrama is its therapeutic value. Psychodrama produces peak experiences—or exciting modes of acting—that often result in individual and social change. In this context, there are a number of basic characteristics of psychodrama that can be delineated as producing these positive results.

There are a variety of therapeutic modalities available to people seeking greater self-awareness toward the goal of resolving their personal and interpersonal problems. The therapeutic process involves relating one's self to a system and interpreting behavior within the terms of a specific methodology. Most therapeutic systems, properly applied, do produce insights, self-awareness, and, consequently, therapeutic progress. The difference between psychodrama and most other methodologies, however, is that psychodrama comes *closest* to the natural scenarios of people in everyday life. This psychodramatic reality factor is, of course, a vital part of pure psychodrama and, as will be demonstrated, can be utilized as a valuable adjunct to other therapeutic modalities.

In psychodrama a person is encountering his conflicts and psychic pain in a setting that more closely approximates his real-life situation than in most other therapeutic approaches. A young man in conflict with a parent talks directly to a person as an auxiliary ego playing his parent. His fantasy (or reality) of his hostility or love can be acted out on the spot. He can experience his pain (in one context, his "primal emotions") not in an artificial setting but in direct relationship to the "father," "mother," or other person who helped build the pain into him, since his enactment takes place as closely as possible to the pertinent, specific core situations in his life.

The resolution of his pain or conflict does not necessarily require an extensive analysis or discussion because he is experiencing the emotions *in situ,* in action. Often when someone has had a deep psychodramatic experience, there is no need for lengthy group discussion—sharing—or analysis. The protagonist has learned about the mystery of his problem in action; he feels better immediately, and it is not necessary to go beyond that point.

People develop problems, conflicts, and psychic pain in the normal course of their day-to-day life scenarios. To be sure, extensive one-to-one or discussion group therapies help to unravel a person's emotional mystery; however, at some point the person involved must enact his discoveries or insights in life. The logic of psychodrama is that the person and the group learns or relearns best in action that most closely approximates life—and that is in psychodrama. In many cases, the combination of individual counseling or verbal group therapy in concert with psychodrama maximizes therapeutic results.

Another important aspect of psychodrama is that it is a mirror of life, not only for the central protagonist or star having a session but for the group present at a session. For the star, the real world is slowed down and the time can be taken to explore critical emotional issues by acting out key life scenes. The enactment of such significant scenarios often helps to resolve problems and provides a clearer perspective on life. In most sessions, benefits can accrue to members of the group other than the central protagonist. Group participants are encouraged to witness aspects of their own lives that became manifest in the session, as if watching a dramatic play that projects their own behavior onto the stage in front of them.

This kind of personal participation either as a protagonist or member of a group in a live psychodrama produces maximum emotional impact. In this same context of identifying with a problem being presented before a group, I believe that you can benefit from reading about a psychodrama session if you allow yourself to participate in the session through personally identifying with the central protagonist. By attempting to become personally involved through identifying as closely as possible with the "stars" and peak scenes in the scenarios of sessions presented throughout the book, I believe the reader can personally benefit from psychodrama.

I have attempted to maximize this emotional experience and benefit by providing detailed descriptions of the meaning and impact of the psychodramatic protocols presented. In brief, therefore, although this book is not primarily intended as a self-help document, if you consciously attempt to involve yourself in the dynamics of the psychodramatic processes and the sessions presented here, you can personally benefit from the experience through the enlargement of your emotional and social perspective.

The starting point for your participation is by reflecting on the inner monodramas that you have going on in your mind at varying times; and then attempting to relate your personal session to those presented here. Your contemplative process, or monodrama, for solving interpersonal problems is apt to be most active when you are encountering some conflict or problem in your life. In this regard, people who have a continuing emotional problem tend to have this inner process going on nonstop until their frustration, conflict, or problem is solved.

In this inner monodrama, many people play all of the roles related to their core-significant problem or issue. For example, in a conflict with your spouse or your parents, you say your lines in some form, then you take their role and answer yourself. You may have someone in mind or conjure someone up to help you tell your antagonist off. This defender is like a defensive double helping you in the conflict. Some people have developed an ability for resolving life problems or conflicts in the confines of their personal monodrama. For most people, however, personal problems are seldom resolved in private reverie, because in your monodrama, without outside help, you are usually restricted to seeing the same sides of an issue. In an actual psychodrama, the relevant others are activated; and in reading about a session, you can better understand how "others" (e.g., parents, spouses, lovers, children) in other people's lives respond.

Obviously, not everyone attempts to resolve their problems on their own in their monodramas. They work out solutions to their problems and conflicts by objectifying their inner-drama through acting out in life or discussion with a close friend or a therapist.

Many people do not have the resources of a therapist or a close friend to help them resolve their inner conflict, or, even when they do, the problem continues. In many cases, psychodrama is a viable alternative. The psychodrama process enables the protagonist to present his internal drama more objectively, with greater clarity; and it often leads to an effective solution. In the psychodramatic process there exists a greater potential for resolution because a group is present. In psychodrama members of the group are called upon as auxiliary egos to play the roles of the others in the interpersonal problem required by the protagonist to explore and solve.

My first psychodrama, over twenty-five years ago, was a memorable event. I did not become the protagonist in the session, but, as a member of the group, I was called upon to become an auxiliary ego by Dr. Moreno, who directed the session. My retrospective presentation and analysis will reveal some of the basic concepts, dynamics, and terminology of a session and, in some measure, will serve as a guide for your participation in psychodrama.

I first met Dr. Moreno in 1949, when I was a graduate student in sociology at New York University and had enrolled in his seminar on psychodrama. Because of Moreno's reputation, charisma, and dramatic approach to teaching, it was one of the most popular courses at the university. Most of Moreno's class sessions were dialectic discussions, but he invited the class, as part of the course, to attend sessions at his Psychodrama Theatre, then on Park Avenue in New York City.

The evening I attended my first psychodrama session, I had a limited idea of what to expect. I had heard Moreno lecture and had read some material on psychodrama; I thought I would see a play—a human drama spontaneously produced by the group on stage.

The psychodrama theater I entered was about fifty by fifty feet. There was a round stage at one end that dominated about a third of the room. The group present consisted of forty people, mostly students, all nervously awaiting the opening of the session.

All attention focused on Dr. Moreno, who appeared suddenly from the wings like a magician. He stood quietly in the center of the stage for several minutes, simply surveying the group. He had a happy-omnipotent look on his beaming face. He was a man of average height, stout, and attired in a corduroy jacket with leather-patched sleeves. Although he stood silently on the stage for two to three minutes, his presence seemed to produce emotional waves. I observed some people in the group flash broad smiles that seemed to speak acceptance. Mingled with this response appeared to be several nervous individuals who looked frightened. Would this mysterious man expose their humiliating self-doubts and secrets? A few were hostile, whispering that Moreno "looked like a clown, a charlatan." Obviously, I had no clear way of knowing whether there was any truth in my perceptions of the group's response. My observations might have been my personal projections onto this charismatic, fascinating man.

He began the session by describing the stage he stood on as a vehicle for expressing all of the heavenly and hellish feelings that existed in the group. He pointed out the difference between the vehicle of the stage as infinite life-space compared to the static nature of the chair in usual therapy. The person acting out his dilemma in psychodrama would encounter "live" all of the people necessary to present his problem. He would not be restricted to simply talking about his problem one-dimensionally. He could act out with members of the group portraying the characters necessary for his essential life scenes.

The people who filled the subject's requirements in the production of a scene were identified as auxiliary egos. Moreno looked at me and said, "For example, if this young man were to act out his conflict with his mother, the lady who portrayed his mother would be an auxiliary ego." I asked Moreno how he knew I had conflict with my mother. He puckishly replied, "Who doesn't?" I soon discovered that acting omniscient and clairvoyant was part of the character of being a psychodrama director. This posture seemed to infuse the group with a sense that the director knew all and facilitated a certain hypnotic quality.

Moreno walked over to a young couple who seemed intrigued by his preliminary performance. "Are you two married?" The young lady beamed, "Not yet, we're engaged." She held up the hand that displayed the diamond ring, symbol of engagement and a characteristic of marital intent for a proper young middle-class couple from Brooklyn.

Moreno took the young lady's hand and brought her on stage. "How would you like a marriage pre-test? Let's explore your compatibility with this charming groom." The young lady assented.

She produced several scenes. With the presentation of each episode, I became more and more intrigued and involved with the drama. In my personal past, I had been there myself with several girls, and the session struck a chord in my own emotional life. Moreno, apparently aware of my intense involvement, selected me to play the auxiliary ego role of her betrothed. I rapidly absorbed the role. In several scenes, I became Phil, a young law student from a proper, reasonably wealthy orthodox family. We enacted several scenes. In the first, I met this beauty, Selma, at a Hadassah dance. In the role, I quickly ascertained she was a virginal princess. Her family background was perfect for me in the role of Phil. As Phil I was a business administration major at New York University. My potential father-in-law owned a large business and as Phil I became consumed with the thought of acquiring a significant piece of my "father-in-law's" wealth when I became the husband of his only child-daughter. In one scene, the father and I coyly discussed the possibility.

An hour into the session, we were sailing toward a perfect marriage. Then an emotional storm erupted—much to my surprise, but not Moreno's.

We were playing the scene in which we were purchasing my intended's engagement ring. Suddenly, this quiet, acquiescent girl ripped the real ring off her finger and threw it at me. "I don't want you—my parents want you but I don't." I asked, "What did I do wrong?" "It's nothing you did, it's what you are. You're exactly like my father. I don't want my mother's life. It's dull and meaningless. That's what I would have with you!"

Moreno then guided her through several scenes that revealed her distaste for the conventional. It became apparent that she was simply following, on the surface, the least line of resistance to her parents, her culture, in accepting in that context this "perfect" young man.

Her inner self craved a more soulful life of creativity. She had a deep, sincere aspiration to become an artist. The session unleashed her inner reality, which conflicted sharply with her external acceptance and presentation of self.

When she *actually* threw the diamond ring at me across the psychodrama stage, the group, and especially her real boyfriend, Phil, were shocked. Deep sobs began to convulse her body. A young lady played her *double*. (A double is someone who helps the protagonist express his or her feelings by physically and emotionally identifying with them.) The double put her arms around the girl and sobbed with her. The emotional, primal response went on for almost five minutes, and Moreno let the catharsis of her emotions take place without interruption. Her lament was, "It's always been this way since I can remember. They only love me when I am the way they want me to be. When I want to be myself, they reject me."

When the girl seemed to be drained of her emotion and pain, Moreno ended the role-playing phase of the session. He sat the couple down at his side and they began to talk about their relationship, as they never had before. There was a deluge of honesty and emotional catharsis. The girl told her intended how she knew he only wanted her for the status and affluence her father could confer on him. The young man admitted this, but also told her how her display of spontaneous fire in the session turned on feelings he never knew he had for her. "I never saw this other side of you before."

Moreno pointed out how they had both colluded in relating to each other's images; that now, with this breakthrough in communication through psychodrama, they might possibly relate to the real other. And it was only through relating to the authentic other person that their relationship had a chance. He pointed out that they could live out their lives with others as robot-images but that now they might relate with greater passion to each other's true selves.

The session produced emotional shock waves in the group. Others began to reveal their identification with a similar problem. Some talked about false relationships that they had with parents rather than spouses. A couple married for twelve years began to talk about the fact that they were right then a horrible example of the fate this young couple might have averted through their psychodrama. They began to detail where they went wrong and discussed how they might become more feeling, authentic, and intimate.

My own reaction was intense. I began to examine my relationships, but more than that: *in playing that young man's role, I became him.* It was my first session as an auxiliary ego, but I realized that the roles I could play in sessions were unlimited, far beyond the roles portrayed by any stage or movie actor. Since that 1949 conversion to psychodrama, I have had the deep and varied experience of enacting almost every role in Western civilization. I have played a priest, a rabbi, Adolf Eichmann, God, a pimp, a psychopathic killer, Jack Ruby, a woman, a homosexual, President Kennedy, etc. The enactment of these roles in psychodrama, in interaction with real people and their problems, has enlarged my existence, a side effect of all sessions.

After Moreno settled the couple down, with positive feedback from him and the group, he gave a long lecture on the elements of psychodrama. The essential ideas he analyzed in the post-discussion introduced me to the basics of the psychodramatic method and its rules.

He emphasized that it was more valuable for the protagonist to act out conflicts than to talk about them. The presentation of relevant others in the protagonist's life represented by auxiliary egos gives a greater sense of reality to the production. The stage, lighting, and props (tables, chairs, etc.) help toward the creation of a greater reality and depth than simply talking in the first person.

Moreno then emphasized his concept of psychodrama in the "here and now." The protagonist always acts in the present tense, even if the scene revolves around a childhood incident. Whenever the protagonist would slip and say in a scene from the past, "When I was five I loved my mother," Moreno would correct the protagonist, "I *am* five and I love my mother." In explaining the "here and now" in psychodrama, Moreno emphasized that a person can never again act in the past. All anyone can do is give their *current* conception of a past situation. Psychodrama enables a person to objectify (in the immediate situation) a significant memory of an important event carried in the psyche.

In psychodrama, a protagonist has complete control over the truth as they see and feel it. For example, a protagonist may *perceive* his mother as overwhelming and oppressive. When the group meets the actual mother, they are surprised to see a quiet, shy person. The session, however, revolves around the protagonist's perception. The protagonist is entitled to his personal perspective on the truth. Later in a session, the reality of other people's viewpoints may be presented, but the protagonist is first entitled to his session—as he sees it.

In a session with someone severely disturbed who sees "a devil," the director and the group do not try to argue him out of what he sees by saying, "You're hallucinating." They join him in his distortion by doubling with him. The group and the director enter the protagonist's world with him, even though at a later session they may attempt to introduce the consensual reality of the group present or the larger societal viewpoint. According to Moreno, "The person's enactment of their reality comes first—their retraining comes later." In this regard, Moreno advocates allowing the protagonist as much as possible to pick *his* scene, *his* place, and *his* auxiliary ego in order to enact *his* problem.

It is an assumption of psychodrama that a protagonist learns and relearns more effectively when they are deeply involved in a crucial scene from their life than if they simply talk about a situation. It involves "insight in action." Often the protagonist who has experienced the insight may experience it on a subconscious level. When this happens, it is usually unnecessary for him to have to verbalize his insight or catharsis. It is his, he has already experienced it in action. As Moreno stated, "Even when an interpretation of an act is made, the action is more primary. There can be no meaningful interpretation without the act taking place first."

There are three phases to a psychodrama session: (1) the warm-up, (2) the action, and (3) the post-discussion. The warm-up and the action of a session are vital; however, the post-discussion is also highly significant. This is the portion of a session during which the group *shares* their empathy and experiences with the protagonist. For example, in the session revolving around the engagement, many members of the group revealed their own uncertainties about accepting the boundaries of marriage. This has the honest effect of apprising the protagonist that he or she is not alone in the dilemma. It also provides the group members with the opportunity to reflect openly about their involvement in the session and to synthesize their responses. There is ample room for analysis in psychodrama, but the basic principle is that analysis should always follow the action and the post-discussion. In the post-discussion phase, the director must draw from the group their identification with the protagonist. This process produces group insight, increases cohesion, and enlarges inter-personal perceptions.

The significance and primacy of the group in psychodrama was a lesson Moreno reiterated throughout my early training with him. Another emphasis was the "act-hunger," the need in people to act beyond or at least in consort with their verbalizations and inner thoughts. Moreno's admonitions to utilize the group's power in action on behalf of a protagonist has been a guiding theme in every psychodrama I have directed over the years.

These themes are illustrated in a session I directed with a lady who could not resolve her conflict in her own monodrama and found no resolution through private verbal encounters with an individual therapist. Her session further delineates how group psychodrama works and, to some degree, how you can participate in a psychodrama scenario by identifying with the protagonist.

The woman's problem has some unique characteristics, but generally it deals with a normal problem that almost everyone experiences at some point in their life: the inability to honestly and openly communicate with a parent. The session provides some insight into the process of externalizing a protagonist's inner monodrama in a situation in which acting out the problem in real life was blocked for rational reasons.

The protagonist had been in a form of counseling therapy where she had in many sessions verbalized her problem on a one-to-one basis. As she put it: "I've talked about my feelings ad nauseum and it has not helped me." She also admitted that she had a monodrama going on in her mind that plagued her and defied resolution on her own. She was fixated on the problem and was seldom able to concentrate on other matters going on in her life.

The forty-year-old woman named Helen comes forward onto the psychodrama stage and begins to warm up to a session by exposing her inner drama to the group. She soliloquizes: "I keep reviewing over and over in my mind something I want to tell my mother. She's in the hospital with terminal cancer. I can't think of anything else. There are some things I feel compelled to tell her while she's still alive. She's very important to me. I hate her and I love her. I hate her because she's dominated my life and I've permitted it. I married a man I didn't love because I knew he was the kind of man she wanted me to marry. I love her because she has always given to me and at times was very good to me. Lately, I think about her constantly. In my mind I tell her off. This makes me feel guilty. So then I tell her how much I love her. In spite of this, when I'm with her I don't actually express any of my feelings. I feel it would be cruel to impose my problems on her at this time. After all, she is dying. I can't hurt her, yet I have this anger in me, and it's just eating me up."

Psychodramatically, we have Helen visit her mother in the hospital. We have someone from the group come up on stage as an auxiliary ego and assume the role of Helen's mother. Helen begins to sob and tells her "mother" in the session how much she loves her and is going to miss her when she's gone. She can express her love, but she is unable to express her hostile feelings. She interrupts the session and says, "How can I tell a dying woman about all of the frustration and hatred she has created in me during my lifetime?"

As the director of the session, I tell Helen, "Of course, in reality we would not want you to do this to your real mother. But this lady here, obviously, is playing your mother, she isn't your mother. Let's psychodramatically explore the size and shape of your hostility—for your sake. Obviously, you can't hurt your mother because she really isn't here. I would strongly urge you to get these feelings out in the open. I've seen hundreds of sessions in which people carry the burden of these festering feelings with them all of their lives because they were unable to act them out. These unexpressed unresolved emotions can be a psychologically painful albatross."

Helen agrees and becomes further mesmerized into the psychodrama. She accepts the auxiliary ego as her mother. She says in one situation she was so angry she wanted to hit her mother. She emotionally gets into the mood of the situation. She is twenty-five. The auxiliary ego mother is denouncing her for the way she looks. She ridicules her for having aspirations for becoming an actress. She tells her she's not that good looking and should grab the first man she can get. Helen gets into the mood of the scene. Her anger builds. We give her a battoca, a foam rubber "weapon" used in group therapy to express hostility. She begins to angrily strike a small table in front of the "mother" auxiliary ego with the battoca, and, combined with the process of her physical violent action, she tells her mother the pain and humiliation she has received all her life from her. Among other epithets she hurls at her, she calls her an "oppressive crazy woman."

Now that Helen has externalized her formerly suppressed inner monodrama, in which for the first time she openly and forcefully expressed her enormous hatred, she begins to cry. "In spite of everything," she sobs to her "mother," "I love you and want you to live." Now that she has expressed her hatred she can express her love, and she does this by tenderly embracing her psychodramatic "mother" in the session. For two hours we explore psychodramatically other aspects of her relationship to her mother in core scenes of their life together. We go back to significant scenes in her childhood, and we now psychodramatically prepare her to face the future.

To prepare her for the inevitable, we have her mother die psychodramatically. We lower the lights in the psychodrama theater. The group present becomes the mourners at the mother's funeral, and Helen delivers a clear and eloquent eulogy (including some of her bitterness) that clarifies and articulates her feelings about her mother and their lifelong relationship.

Other members of the group, both men and women, emotionally identify with her psychodramatic portrait of her mother. Several come forward and briefly enact and verbalize their emotions about their own mothers. Their responses in this session that are summarized here reflect only a few of the broad array of attitudes I have heard expressed in hundreds of other sessions on this theme:

"I forgive you, Mother, for all the terrible things you inflicted on me, because I now understand all the crap you took from Dad."

"I will always hate you—you always were an insufferable bitch. I'm glad you're dead. I feel relieved not to have you in my head all the time telling me what to do. I feel happy and free for the first time in my life."

"Mother, I only have one complaint, why did you always force religion on me? I don't believe all that nonsense about heaven and hell. And there is no God. If there were, why did He let the little kids in Vietnam get napalmed? I miss you, but certainly not your unbearable preaching."

"I feel lost without you. You were a beautiful person, someone I could always turn to. Especially when I was a kid, you were always right there for me. I don't understand how others can have this hostility for their mothers. You were a wonderful mother and I really miss you."

Helen, as the central protagonist of the session, was very intrigued with each vignette presented by every other member of the group who came forward. She said that she felt relieved to know that some of them shared her own feelings.

A few days after the session, Helen visited her mother in the hospital. The following week in the group she said: "The session and my last visit to my mother have lifted an enormous burden from my mind. I feel completely different about her. I could talk to her for the first time without guilt, pain, or anger. The session clarified my emotions and I felt freer to honestly talk to her. I believe I'm able to say goodbye to her now without rancor. Also, now that my mind is free from that pain and frustration, I can focus on other more positive things in my life."

One basis for psychodrama enactment, as in Helen's session, is that the person cannot act out the problem in real life—for rational and sometimes irrational reasons. The psychodramatic situation provides a safe, controlled, and beneficial opportunity for exploring the protagonist's inner drama with other people present who, invariably, can relate to the problem from their own experience. Among its other attributes, psychodrama provides an opportunity to rehearse for the actual life situation. In any case, the constant replay of a person's inner monodrama on such issues as a sense of inadequacy, dealing with rejection, feelings of envy or hostility, or other personal problems is usually a fruitless search. Also, for many people certain problems are not resolved by simply talking them out in one-to-one verbal therapy sessions. In psychodrama, however, when the vectors and structure of problems are objectified through the help of other people in action in a psychodramatic theater of life, these matters can often be effectively resolved.

Many people, after their first participation in psychodrama, raise the question, "Isn't it painful to enact a difficult experience even in the controlled environment of a psychodrama?" Sometimes it is, but the basic premise of the question is not accurate. *It is impossible to exactly relive any experience.* What is usually produced in psychodrama is the person's *here-and-now* mental picture of an important past scenario of his life. The concept of the *here and now* in psychodrama thus encompasses past and future projections of significant life events as they currently exist in the person's internal monodrama.

An important aspect of psychodrama is that all of these time states are explicated in action. Some of these issues are revealed in the case example of a series of psychodrama sessions I ran with a young man incarcerated in a state hospital for the so-called criminally insane. Ralph, at eighteen, was in custody for blacking out of control and attempting to kill his father. He almost succeeded. The verbal interactions he had with various therapists in the hospital about his "past behavior" (which we learned through psychodrama was constantly on his mind) had admittedly been of limited help in reaching him. His immediate therapist had participated in several psychodrama sessions and requested that I direct a session with Ralph to help him explore some of Ralph's psychodynamics in action. Ralph's therapist was present at all of the sessions and very productively followed the leads we produced in our psychodramas into his private therapeutic verbal sessions with Ralph. In this case, psychodrama became a valuable adjunct to Ralph's individual therapy.

In addition to Ralph's potential for violence, another symptom that he manifested was a body tic. When it was active, his body would writhe in an epileptic fashion. The tic usually seemed to appear whenever he felt anger or was under pressure. According to a medical report by a doctor who had examined Ralph, there appeared to be no physiological basis for the tic. In the first psychodrama session I ran with Ralph as the protagonist, I noted that the tic was enacted and accentuated whenever there was reference to his father, or sometimes even when the word *father* was used.

In the session, Ralph led us back to a basic and traumatic scene in his life with his father. He acted out a horrendous situation that occurred when he was eight: his father punished him by tying him up by his hands to a ceiling beam in their cellar—like meat on a hook—and then beat him with a belt.

We determined from several sessions with Ralph, and my consultations with his therapist, that the traumatic experience of the whipping and other parental atrocities produced his tic, because the tic appeared after this particular beating and, as indicated, there did not seem to be any physiological basis for it. The tic seemed to be a way he controlled striking back at his basic antagonist, his father. In brief, Ralph had two extreme postures that emerged from his parental abuse: one was the tic that incapacitated him from the other—extreme, uncontrolled violence. Other sessions revealed that his rage toward his father was often displaced onto others, especially other children at school.

(In relating Ralph's plight, it is apparent that the parental abuse he was subjected to and his symptomatic response were of epic proportions. It is important to bear in mind that "the battered-child syndrome" is both physical and emotional and *is a matter of degree*. Although very few children are exposed to the extreme abuse that Ralph was, many [both boys and girls] have experienced some level of this type of negative socialization and have developed symptoms of rage, personality postures, and self-destructive tendencies in direct relationship to the negative causal factors in their life. In my work in psychodrama, I have seen many levels of intensity and patterns of Ralph's parental syndrome in people who, for the most part, are normal functioning members of society.)

The father, who had Ralph hospitalized, was obviously the arch object of Ralph's hatred. Ralph could seldom talk to his father in life. He would either manifest the incapacitating tic, run away, or, as he finally did, attempt to kill him.

In the final scene of one psychodrama, we had progressed to a point where he accepted a male nurse as an auxiliary ego in the role of his father. In the psychodrama scene, Ralph would alternately produce the tic or attempt to attack his "father." There was hardly any verbalization of Ralph's rage—he required an action form to express his emotions—and the time factor was in the psychodramatic "here and now" that included varied time frames.

After Ralph had physically acted out much of his rage, I finally improvised a psychodramatic vehicle that facilitated a conversation between Ralph and his auxiliary ego "father." I put a table between him and his "father." At the same time he talked to his father, I gave him the option and the freedom to punch a pillow that he accepted symbolically as his father. This combination of psychodrama devices enabled Ralph to structure in thought and put into words his deep venom for his father. He blurted out much of his long-repressed hatred in a lengthy diatribe. Finally, we removed the props, and after his rage was spent, he fell into his "father's" arms and began to sob, "Why couldn't you love me? I was really a good kid, Dad. Why couldn't you love me?"

Although he went through several phases of his hostility in several sessions, he could not go all the way and *forgive his father,* a symbolic act that I have determined from many sessions would help to relieve him of the ball of hostility in his gut that produced his violent acting-out behavior.

In a later session, we had him play the role of his father, and he for the first time began to empathize with the early experiences in his father's life that brutalized him. Ralph's grandfather—who beat his son—was the original culprit and Ralph was indirectly receiving the fallout of his father's anger toward his father, or Ralph's grandfather. When Ralph reversed roles and returned to himself, it diminished his hostility towards his father and he, at least psychodramatically, that day forgave him.

All of the material acted out in the psychodrama sessions was more closely examined in his private sessions with his therapist. Also, I had a number of productive discussions with both Ralph and his therapist on an individual basis. This combination of therapeutic activity seemed to be most effective in helping Ralph solve his emotional problems. In my follow-up of Ralph's case, I learned that he had made a reasonable adjustment after leaving the hospital. He stayed clear of his father because he couldn't fully handle that relationship. The positive results were that he went to work, married at twenty, and, according to the reports I received, for the most part adjusted to a law-abiding life.

A central point in explicating Ralph's extreme psychodrama experience is to reveal that the learning-in-action on his part, combined with his private sessions, was effective. Ralph could not just *talk* about his anger. He required a vehicle such as psychodrama that gave him the opportunity to physically and psychologically reenact the scenarios of the early parental crimes against him in their bizarre details. In my experience with psychodrama, this seems to be the case for most people. Although most people's problems are not as extreme as Ralph's, at times we all require an action-oriented psychodramatic experience for catharsis from and insight into an emotional problem.

Most people require an active vehicle for expression, either exclusively or as an adjunct to an individual-verbal approach. It is apparent to many individual therapists that many clients, when embroiled in the discussion of deep emotions, either have the urge or actually get up off the therapeutic couch or chair and begin to physically move around. It is precisely at this point of action that psychodrama comes into play. There is no real conflict between verbal analysis and role-playing; there is, however, ample psychodramatic evidence that most people could benefit from some form of learning-in-action as an adjunct to their verbal-discussion therapy.

A protagonist who flourished in a combination of psychodrama and individual therapy after several years of moderate progress in a strictly individual talk therapy made the following observations on the necessity of an action method in her life:

"I went to several shrinks. I must admit I learned a lot, but I also found it frustrating. When I would get into the anger that I turned on myself in the form of depression, I wanted to scream and break things. But there I would sit on my hostility.

"One of my therapists had an office full of fine furniture, plants, and antiques. The scene totally militated against my really expressing my anger. If I blew up, like I have many times in psychodrama, I would have busted up several thousand dollars' worth of furniture. I might pour coffee or break an ashtray on his Oriental carpet.

"Also I couldn't yell or scream because of the people in the outer office. So I sat there like a good polite little patient talking about my depression, which never went away until I opened up in psychodrama."

We have determined from many psychodrama sessions that depression is a common feeling and is the symptom of many people's underlying problem of unexpressed rage. The depression is essentially related to the containment of frustrations in one's self. The depression often results precisely from withholding feelings of anger and hostility—a condition that is often exacerbated by some therapeutic situations in which the person is allowed only to talk.

Psychodrama in either its classic form or as an adjunct to verbal therapy provides the action vehicle for experiencing the size and shape of hostile and other emotions in a personalized setting in which the object of one's venom is not physically hurt. In the extreme, "killing" someone psychodramatically (as Ralph did in one of his sessions) can provide the opportunity to act out and exorcise a deep feeling of hatred without anyone actually becoming the physical victim of the aggression. Another advantage of acting out aggression in psychodrama is that the protagonist can do it in—a form of cinematic slow motion—thus enabling him to understand the experience and learn from it in each frame of the action. Moreover, in psychodrama we often use a form of instant replay, until the protagonist feels he has properly explored his emotions; we can then have him experience one or more different and appropriate modes of action in the same situation.

Another important aspect of an action method such as psychodrama is that protagonists can see for themselves and learn from the action of other protagonists enacting scenarios that parallel their own life experiences. In psychodrama you are not verbally told a story; you can see the epic scenes of the other person's scenario and can vicariously benefit from the action. You can see that others face conflicts and dilemmas very much like your own. This very visible perception of a problem is often parallel to participating in your personal drama being enacted on stage.

People who are ordinarily reluctant to open up in a group situation are often spurred into action and awareness by an intense psychodrama session because of the visual drama. Sometimes an element of overacting is encouraged. The psychodramatic session may have characteristics of what Moreno has called "surplus reality." A situation is blown up out of proportion and magnified to enable the subject and the group to get a closer look at it under the psychodramatic microscope. The subject and the group get to see themselves with all of their facades, in a setting in which errors of judgment and behavior are not as destructive or traumatic as they might be if acted out in the real situation. These surplus-reality explorations have the after-effect of providing you with new ways to be more creative, inventive, and spontaneous in your actual human relationships.

This action awareness and insight does not manifest itself in the same way in individual or even talk or encounter group therapies. In these forms of interaction, the person *tells* his story. But when a protagonist acts out his psychodrama in front of a group, every (unverbalized) nuance of body posture and movement reveals aspects of his life that would not appear in the one-dimensional verbal presentation. Psychodrama, like good theater, has the set, the movement, and the dialogue all presented in tandem in their live context.

Psychodramatic scenarios, therefore, not only mirror life but also reflect existence in its many complex dimensions. Reacting to the psychodramatic experience is parallel in some ways to observing a fine drama in the theater. One difference, however, between theater and psychodrama is that theater, with all of its magnetism and dramatic impact, unlike psychodrama, has a predictability about the characters and the flow of the drama. Most dramatic plays or movies have standard plots or are set forms. *Hamlet* is always *Hamlet*. *Cabaret* remains *Cabaret,* and the dialogue of *Death of a Salesman* is seldom altered.

There is a great variety in psychodrama sessions, and there often emerges a unique and sudden twist in the plot or an irony that is more apt to occur in life than in theater. There are parallels between psychodrama sessions because material is drawn from the same basic culture; however, no two psychodrama sessions are ever substantially the same. In psychodrama, there are as many variations and curlicues of life as in life itself. This is the case because psychodrama sessions penetrate beyond the surface of one-dimensional dialogue or performance into the myriad and complex aspects of human behavior. Dreams, fantasies, religious emotions, sexual fantasies, feelings, and communication with dead people can all be part of a psychodramatic production.

Brilliant dramas, such as Arthur Miller's *Death of a Salesman* or Shakespeare's *Hamlet,* certainly get beneath the skin of life, but psychodrama has one dimension that does not exist, even in the most profound theatrical production. In psychodrama Willy Loman *is* Willy Loman, Macbeth *is* Macbeth, Cyrano *is* Cyrano. The protagonist is not play-acting; the acting flows from a real person who is presenting himself and the scenarios of his peak life experiences.

Another important aspect of psychodrama is the element of

flexibility and spontaneity. A play must follow the dramatic sequence set by the play's author. In psychodrama we can select key scenes, change dialogue on the spot, follow new emotional trails that emerge, speed up or slow the action down, or simply stop (freeze-frame) and focus on crucial situations or scenes. These possibilities enable a psychodrama group to give proper time and emphasis to the most significant aspects of a person's life scenarios.

Psychodrama provides a unique acting-out possibility in a concrete form for portraitures of many social roles. A person in psychodrama can, either as a protagonist, a double for the star, an auxiliary ego, or as a member of the group present, identify with or act out the infinite roles of his culture, and learn in the process. In psychodrama a child can become a parent, a husband can become a wife, a white person becomes a black person, a young person becomes old, a woman can become a man, and vice versa. The possibilities are as many, varied, and complex as the myriad roles in a given society. The experience goes beyond identifying with a superb theatrical performer or empathizing with another. Participating in the psychodramatic process tends to facilitate the expansion of a person's role repertoire so that everyone can learn more precisely in action what it is like to be another person in another role. *Being* in this way in psychodrama can help resolve a personal problem, but a more general impact can be the enhancement of communication and compassion in the larger society. Beyond sociological analysis, which tells what human experience is, the psychodramatic process provides the opportunity for you to experience life in a variety of new situations, and to experiment with new responses to old situations. Also beyond therapy, the existential state that your imagination can only hint at in fantasy can become an emotional reality in psychodrama.

Psychodramatic theater does not only focus on the resolution of specific emotional problems. Sometimes a simple direct session is a microcosmic form of a macrocosmic philosophical issue in a society.

The drama of a "philosophical session" potentially can enlarge a person and the group's philosophical perspective, since the individual's session almost always has broader implications than the protagonist's private psyche. When a psychodrama is dramatically absorbing and entertaining, the session will produce, as does good theater, a profound philosophical impact. In brief, the participants in an ideal psychodrama session, in addition to having a specific problem or conflict resolved, can be entertained and have their philosophical perspective on life enlarged. Participation for therapy or the resolution of a problem, therefore, is not the only, or necessarily the primary, goal of psychodrama.

A classic psychodrama, directed by my wife, Donna, in which I participated as an auxiliary ego provides an example of the many and varied impacts of a psychodrama session that go beyond immediate problem resolution. This session, which led the group present into a broader philosophical perspective, is presented in part to cue you in on how to participate more broadly in the variety of psychodrama scenarios that will be described.

This prototypical "philosophical session" was triggered when Kian, a young Oriental man of thirty, commented in a warm-up discussion, "Here I am, there is only *one* other person in my emotional life. Her name is Paulette and I have not seen her in ten years." The emotional tone of Kian's voice and the unusual implications of his lonely statement were an invitation to a session. Kian quickly revealed by his further comments and demeanor a fierce pride about himself and his heritage. He is melancholy. He begins to talk about how ten years ago he lost Paulette, "the only love I ever had in my life." It is apparent that the specter of Paulette dominates his life—now, ten years later. As he warms up to the session, it becomes apparent to the group that his immediate sexual fantasies, his career, his celibacy, his mood are all related to this haunting lady from the past and the meaning of his memory and dreams about her in his life.

He acts out several scenes with the help of auxiliary egos, who play the necessary roles. The session ran for two hours. The essential scenes of the psychodrama are presented here in summary form.

Scene I: He meets Paulette at college and begins to date her on a steady basis for over six months. They are both twenty. He falls in love with her, and he assumes by her response that his attraction to and feelings about her are mutual and are reciprocated.

Scene II: He is with a childhood friend who is visiting him at the university, and he takes him to the woman's dormitory where Paulette lives. He is anxious for his good friend to meet the woman he loves and hopes to marry. He and the friend arrive unannounced in the busy lobby. To Kian's surprise a man at the reception desk who is unknown to him is asking for Paulette's room. The receptionist phones, then tells the stranger Paulette will be right down. Kian stands there spellbound by the painful experience. Paulette appears. She doesn't see Kian, who has moved with his friend to a corner of the lobby. He watches with amazement and is stunned when he sees Paulette leaving with the other man—apparently on a date!

The director instructs me as his double in the scene to join with Kian in the soliloquy of his psychic pain and jealous feelings about what has just happened.

KIAN: "We've been together for a year. I have loved her deeply. All of this time I had no indication of any kind that there was anyone else. I am also extremely embarrassed in front of my friend. I've been telling him what a wonderful girl she is and how much in love we are and how there is no one else for me—and now this! Before this happened I had every intention of marrying her. This destruction of my feelings of honor and pride is insufferable."

SCENE III

After a phone call to her the next day, Kian meets again with Paulette. He is full of anger and self-righteousness, and he won't allow her to explain or even speak. He simply wants revenge and does not permit Paulette to explain her behavior.

KIAN: You really wounded me.

He launches into a diatribe in which he chastises her in every possible way.

PAULETTE: Please let me explain.

KIAN (*full of fury*): No explanation is possible. I don't want to do this, but this is the end of us. Paulette and Kian no longer exist.

Kian reveals to the group that later that evening he seriously considered suicide. His pride would not let him accept the psychic pain of being betrayed. She phones him several times, and he refuses to talk to her. A week later he meets Paulette's roommate in the university cafeteria.

SCENE IV

PAULETTE'S ROOMMATE: Kian, you're incredible. Why wouldn't you let Paulette explain?

KIAN: There's nothing to explain. I saw her and this other person, and that told me the complete story.

Kian reverses roles and plays Paulette's roommate.

KIAN AS PAULETTE'S ROOMMATE: I'll tell you what's to explain. The guy she went out with is my boyfriend. He had tickets to a play, I was ill, and I insisted that she go with him so as not to waste the tickets. She went reluctantly. That's all that happened. Period.

Kian now returns to his own role.

KIAN: Oh, my God! I should have given her a chance to explain.

He begins to sob (in the immediate psychodrama situation). The group present is very empathetic. They ask him what happened when he rushed over to see her? Now she refused to see him no matter what he said. She was apparently deeply hurt by his behavior, which allowed no explanation on her part. She decided that a man who could be that obstinate and implacable was no one to consider for a permanent relationship. Kian attempted to see her again on several occasions, but Paulette now refused to see him. He finally gave up calling her.

Several months after the experience, the school year ended and Paulette, a graduating senior, left the university. When Kian heard she had left, he tried to find her. In fact, he related the many and various ways he tried to find her over a ten-year period.

He thinks of no one else and has looked for her everywhere possible. He indicated that he especially goes to concerts because she was a musician and a lover of music. Over the ten-year search,

Kian mentioned that he went to hundreds of concerts—always looking for Paulette.

SCENE V

Although there are many other complex psychodynamic vectors to Kian's obsessional search, the psychodrama director decides in this session to use a future-projection technique, bringing closure to Kian's pursuit. Donna sets up a scene at a concert where Kian finally "finds" Paulette (played by an auxiliary ego).
KIAN: My God, it's really you.
"PAULETTE": Yes. How are you?
KIAN: Fine. But you don't know how I've missed you and longed for you!
"PAULETTE": The way you acted that last time, I had no idea.

Kian goes on to pour his heart out about his love for her. Even though the real Paulette is not present, we see and feel the depth of his emotions. After he has exhausted these feelings, the director sets up a "consolation prize" scene with several women from the group in turn trying to attract him by parading in front of him and extolling their virtues as possible girlfriends who are "better than Paulette." But he clearly demonstrates his singlemindedness and that his total interest, even now, is for no one but Paulette.

The session at this point has had a profound effect not only on Kian but also on the people present in the psychodrama group. Obviously, Kian had fixated his life; at least his romantic life was curtailed at the age of twenty when he lost Paulette. No other girl has meant anything to him since. The session also revealed the degree to which a person can relate to an image, a memory, or a fantasy that has limited real meaning except in the person's mind.

The director set up a further experimental scene with Kian and "Paulette." He puts his arms around her again and pours out his longing and emotions. He sobs for almost five minutes. After he has expressed his feelings of love, he begins for the first time to examine some of the reality of his fantasy. He begins to question: Are you married now? Maybe you have kids? Are you as beautiful as you were? Maybe you've changed, and maybe I've changed.

In this scene, Kian admits to the group that this was the first time in the ten years of his obsession for Paulette that he has realistically looked at his dream. He further reveals that although he had talked about it many times, to many people, this was the first time the hard walls of his fantasy had been pierced. The ambiance, the total mood of the session, reaches Kian. There is an immediate change in his perspective. Jokingly, he asks the director, "How about getting some of those girls back up here? Maybe I can be attracted to one of them now." All of the girls who were in the prior scene spontaneously return to the stage. He now clearly seems more open to other possibilities. All of the "potential girlfriends" on stage embrace Kian. For the first time in ten years, he begins to respond to women other than Paulette. The group spontaneously reinforces Kian's apparent new openness and response by applauding him as he leaves the stage at the end of the session.

The session had a profound effect on the group. One person present later wrote up his experience:

"Probably one of the best experiences I ever had was with Kian and Paulette. I felt like saying, 'Grab her now! Don't let her get away! To hell with your pride! Let her explain. But that was all in the past.' I am sure, and it came out later, that Kian would handle the situation much differently today. There was a powerful emotional release in the group when Kian found Paulette in the session. The release occurred simultaneously with Kian on stage and in the group. This was the most dramatic and poignant experience I've ever had in my life. Among other reactions, in the post-discussion we all clearly realized that one should come to grips with reality and not go on living a fantasy."

Several weeks later we had further discussions with Kian, not only about the meaning of the session to him but to the group. We discussed the issue of how many people are "in search of Paulette" in a broader philosophical and emotional sense.

Paulette was to Kian, symbolically, something like Rosebud in Orson Welles' film classic *Citizen Kane*. As a young boy, Kane was ripped from his mother and a home he loved that was sym-

bolically represented by his precious sled, Rosebud. After amass-
ing enormous wealth, Kane, in his Hearstlike castle, on his death-
bed whispers his final word, "Rosebud." Nothing he had or could
acquire ever took the place for him of the sweet memories of
love associated in his mind with his early childhood and Rosebud.

One member of the group, deeply affected by Kian's session,
sorted out the meaning of the session to him in the following way:

"I've been married for fifteen years and my life is good. I love
my wife, who is now thirty-five. But I must admit the real love
of my life and the sweetest, most romantic time of my life was
with that twenty-year-old girl who is now my thirty-five-year-old
wife and a much different person. I remember that young, beautiful girl vividly. I remember our romantic and fabulous sexual
relationship. But that twenty-year-old woman, my Paulette, is
gone. She only exists in my memory.

"I love my wife now, but I'm sure part of my current feeling
is related to the fact that in appearance and demeanor she is the
closest person in the world to that twenty-year-old girl, the
'Paulette,' I once loved so passionately and completely."

How many marriages or relationships are held together by the
fact that the immediate spouse resembles the peak experience of
those early times? How many people love their obnoxious fifteen-
year-old child partly because the child resembles the five-year-old
darling he or she used to be? No person or relationship from our
past can ever be fully reproduced in our present consciousness—
even when we have a continuing relationship with the same person. The fact is that they are not the same person, nor are we.

One view of Kian's psychodrama is that clinically here is a man
with a fixed obsession. That is true, and this aspect of his problem
requires attention. But on a broader level, the session should also
be viewed for its philosophical implications that related to the
images and fantasies of life.

There are, no doubt, some distinct emotional differences between participating in actual psychodrama sessions and attempting
to participate in the role of reader in the psychodramatic sce-

narios that will be presented here. Despite this expected difference, I believe it will be useful to you to read the following (unedited) free association chronicle written by a young lady named Susan Hecht, who participated in a series of psychodrama sessions. In my many years of psychodrama practice, I have had hundreds of participants chronicle their emotional responses to sessions. In my view, Susan has most cogently documented her varied reactions to psychodrama and implicitly provided an insightful guide on how to participate in psychodrama.

Susan is in her mid-twenties, quite attractive, and is a practicing schoolteacher and poet. She entitled her chronicle "How Psychodrama Affected My Life, or Snow White and the Looking Glass":

> I came into Psychodrama searching for "my self." Actually I really wanted someone to hand me a palatable identity I could swallow without too much trouble, so I could continue with my life in a sensitive and sensible manner. The psychodrama group offered no second-hand identities for sale. It did become a mirror, a place I could identify with others and see myself. It offered me a vehicle to look within the past and see how it still fucks up my present. This is a confessional about what I saw, felt, learned and thought these past ten Fridays. It is written in a journal form, although all the entries are condensed and run together for cohesiveness.

> There is a husband and wife team conducting the group: Donna and Lewis Yablonsky. He reminds me of my cousin; blond, a little round and cozy-warm, sarcastic sometimes. Donna starts the class off with some explanations of Psychodrama. I like to watch her, she seems ethereal with an air of fineness about her that models have. She is, alas, human and croaks tonight because of a cold in her throat. We all introduce ourselves. I have a hard time remembering my name. This happens more and more to me lately and makes me quite nervous. I was nervous anyway before class but trying to be open to the girl next to me. She doesn't think the group is for her. Already! It's only been 14 minutes! She says she is just "out of analysis" and is afraid of "being hurt and opened without being closed again." I know she is referring to her emotional self, but the process sounds like surgery to me.

I figure that I hurt so much already, any opening of my sores will be a relief, and if I'm not put back together, well, what experiences in my life have put me back together? The introduction isn't much, mainly terms to help us identify the technique. I space a lot trying to think of ways to be open and friendly for the first time in my life.

I remember the sessions most of all, and that first session with Jeff is anything but dull. Jeff is small-boned and fragile looking for a man of 31. Dark-haired, conservatively dressed, like an ivy-league college student with shirt, vest and patent leather shoes. But, he never wears socks so I know he is a rebel at heart. He admits to "being under analysis" and having troubles breaking the umbilical cord from his parents.

Lewis and Jeff start talking about the problem Jeff has with his parents. His mother has remarried and has her own career as a model; his father is a French casanova, promising him everything but never delivering the Arpège. Jeff had been carted off to military schools and to his grandparents. He had been sarcastic and stubborn but never aggressive or independent until now. It was hard to break the pattern of wanting their love, their approval, their trust even when he knew there was no other way to grow up.

The session takes him back to his boyhood in military school. He is docile most of the time. He smirks. He acts like he is an obnoxious little kid. I identify. I hate his parents because they remind me of mine, all talk and no touch, no tenderness. Words don't mean a damn thing to a little kid, not a damn thing. We relive various episodes in Jeff's life: his dad promising to visit him, his mother saying she loves him but she is too busy to see him more often. Donna plays his mother and hugs him. Jeff doesn't look too comfortable. It's time for Mother to be out of the picture. Lewis sets the scene so Father is dead and Jeff has to decide whether or not to bring him back to life. I am almost hysterical: Let him die! I think. Let the mother-fucker die and good riddance to all those who are hypocrites, all those who promise empty spoons to suck on. Jeff gives a eulogy that takes almost 20 minutes and brings him up from the dead. I did not understand then, how he could be that forgiving. I am young yet.

In the post-session discussion we all tell how we identify and Linda expresses how she came close to tears (she, too, is in analysis) and goes immediately into a session with her father, and herself. She has an incredible amount of hatred for herself, a quality I thought I cornered the market on. Her father had always put her down and made her feel like a slut. Ugh. I hate lecherous old men, I hate incest. I, apparently, hate a lot. I want to talk to Linda afterward and tell her how I admire her for going up the very first time and exposing the whole rotten past, but I can't, I am too shy. So I go home to hate my closed, shy self in private.

By the time class meets again, I am ready for anything. The week has gone badly and I walk into class 15 minutes late trying hard to look like I am not having a nervous breakdown. I notice right off that Jeff is there and Linda is not. Would she be there if I had said something last Friday? Oh . . . shit. I can't take the blame anymore for everything. Maybe she felt the opening and it hurt too much. At any rate, Lewis is sitting three rows in front of me and smiles hello. Donna is doing something on stage with an empty chair. She asks people to put themselves, emotionally I guess, into the chair and then talk to themselves. A couple of people try and they are emotionally OK, which is neat for them, but very boring for us. I am restless and decide I could use some talking too. I tell Susan what an asshole she is; how disorganized, overweight and hypocritical, and many other adjectives I tell her on a daily basis. Lewis gets excited and moves in for the kill. He starts questioning me about the state of Susan's condition. From what I can see, she is pretty messed up. We decide Susan could use a session. Personally, I think she could use a kick in the pants as well.

I remember my session fairly well. I do not space out or go hysterical. I have things to say, a vendetta to revenge. My mother is the object of my hatred and frustration. I blame her for all my problems and hang-ups. I hate her for all the things she had to say to me that I had never replied to. I hate her because she didn't approve of me being myself, not that I knew who that was, either. I hate her precisely because I don't know who I am, and here I sit at 26, a non-identity. I am sick of my crisis, and Mother receives all the blows for my neuroses. I cry and scream with all the 18 year old fury I can muster up. I hit that god-damned pillow with all the 26 year old sexual fury I can muster up. God, do I hate her for that hour. And then I realize she is a person someone quite different than the one I hate. I realize the person I hate is in me, is, in fact, ME. oh my. revelations. what do I do now. . . .

People come up to me and tell me how they admired me, how I have guts and courage to do that session. I don't see it, really, but I love the attention and compassion. I do see how desperately I want to be admired and loved, how empty and ignored I have felt all my life. Privately I know that it wasn't so much guts that got me up on the stage, as pain. When you hurt so bad, that you've had hives for three months, like I do, then you haven't got a whole lot to lose.

I go home that night and remember my marriage. I was married for seven years to an engineer. I had been 18 and rebellious. I had been a fool. I closed myself off from any honest communication with anybody, even me, and denied any feeling that might get in the way of basic survival. Great parts of me started to die. The effect marriage had on me was the same effect as putting bugs in a bottle without any air holes. We start to climb the walls, we pace a lot, we twitch, and finally, we don't care. I am beginning to put some air holes in the bottle, and am testing them in this group. I remember how Jeff came up and doubled with me. Oh do I love him for that. I didn't know how alone I felt up there until he stood by me, and said what I couldn't say and touched me. I almost cry again just thinking how nice it was to have a friend. Even if I don't know him really there is a bond now. I want to give of myself to others in that group, to share what positive feelings I took away tonight. I write several poems:

> I've established
> one can only go home again
> to peer an eye or two
> over the back fence,
> but no definite cuddling
> is available anymore.

> Regardless of all the dozing
> and dreaming I do,
> I'd like to fly a new kite,
> I'd like to hop right on
> that damn kite's back
> and ride . . .
> I'm tired of putting myself on hold.

By the next week, I am cynical again and have the distinct feeling of having given a good performance. I wonder about becoming an actress, but I've been through this escape before. I really thought I would change after last week, become an extrovert perhaps, but no. Still I am shy and have a hard time carrying on a conversation with anybody. I decide I am tired of performing and want something, anything, to come more naturally. Playing other people's daughters seems to come naturally. Eva has a session and I'm elected to be her daughter. I am pleased to be a part, but a little resentful to be so typecast. I want to be independent and grown-up. What a shuck my life is, I feel, to always be someone's daughter.

Later on, I try to double with Donna, who is acting out her teen-age years. I feel inadequate next to her grace and thinness. She is talking about not feeling pretty enough, about becoming a star. Oh shit, isn't there anyone who has a formula for satisfaction. It never occurs to me how much I identify with Everyone until later, and how much I learn about myself through vicarious experiences.

We play a game called Lifeboat. Seven people go up on stage and pretend they are in the middle of the ocean. They each give a little blurb about why they should survive over everyone else in the boat. Every seven minutes, they cast someone to the sharks. Ethel challenges the sociologist who crosses his legs. Ethel is repetitive at times, but the sociologist is a clam. Bob changes the whole premise and wants to fix the boat. He is the first to go. The ex-actor says, "I want to survive because I'm damned curious." I agree and figure it is that idea, more than anything else in life, that keeps me getting up in the morning. I like him. I like the game and decide to use it at school in my 8th grade Literature and Composition class.

The game goes over extremely well. The students want to know statistics: how big the boat is, what equipment is available, etc., before the game even starts. The audience is vocal and tries to persuade the members of the boat who to cast out.

The two girls with the loudest voices stay alive. The participants all agree they weren't too serious about the game though because they knew it was just a game and kept that in mind. They were open about the reasons they voted against people: he's too heavy and we'll sink, I hate her guts, she's too quiet. If the situation was real, they seemed to agree they would try to find another solution besides throwing people overboard. Kids are cruel sometimes, but not sadistic. We start a whole discussion on survival, the strong vs. the weak, what tools we need to survive in American society, etc.

In our next session, I notice people are in clusters of two and three. Donna is directing and reading a chapter from Lew's manuscript on psychodrama. I listen at times and just watch her at other times. I take a few notes that seem to pertain to me somehow:

—It is important to understand family and sociometric structure to understand delinquency

—Some parents have an invested interest in keeping their kid sick

—Cocoon of fantasy

—Social death: restore losses with new friends, love and spontaneity

—Conserve, a diminished product of creative process: movie, book, technique of role reversal. Problem is tendency to be enslaved by the conserves.

During the reading I also think about my marriage again, and how I want to change my life but don't know how. I think about my love life. How there are too many men of too little substance who distract me but offer little else. How I am incapable of a relationship at this minute, my fear of marriage, of boredom, of social death. I think of an interesting statement that Eva had made to her "mother" during her session that keeps coming back to me. She said, "Why don't you get it (love) your own way. It's not my responsibility anymore." I want to say that to my mother too.

Jean has a session with her son-in-law. I get to play daughter again. This time, I resent it, thoroughly, but I become involved in the part and act totally obnoxious. I am good at that. It is easier to be obnoxious than happy.

Sometime during the next few sessions we do two activities I like and adapt to my classes at work: the magic shop and the social atom. [The *magic shop* is a psychodramatic warm-up game. The director runs a shop that contains everything: money, courage, love, health, etc. The catch is that the group member has to give something of himself for what he wants, with bargaining taking place. The *social atom* involves a person in sketching for the group a diagram of five to ten people who are emotionally important to the person. The person drawing the diagram is placed in the center of his social atom.] By the way, I'm getting to be much more comfortable with directing my kids in role-playing sessions at my school. One girl, Evelyn, role-played telling a boy that she liked him as a friend and not as a boy friend. Another time several students role-played a bad situation they were having with another teacher. In both cases neither problem is actually solved, but the students are allowed to see the problem from more than one viewpoint and are not so nervous or angry anymore, and thus more able to carry on communication. The role-playing also allows me to be an observer or director, and eliminates me from the role of arbitrator, which I, and my hives, appreciate.

We did the Magic Shop in my Group Counseling class at school, which is usually just a rap session for whatever topics the kids bring up. It is a small group, about 19 altogether. We put up on the board subjects like Friendship, Beauty, Courage, and Strength. Jeff, a student, wanted Courage but was unwilling to give up the extra food he eats that makes him overweight. Sharon wanted Friendship but was unwilling to give up the long beautiful nails that scratch her peers or her too loud voice. After a couple of other participants, the majority lost interest. They wanted results, they said, and besides I couldn't give them what they wanted even if they paid the price. They could, I argued, get it themselves. Surely friendship or courage was within their grasp. They sighed and said they couldn't see the point of the game. It was fantasy.

Our Social Atom exercise in the group was 100% positive. I have a Communication class of 15, and we all drew social atoms to help us define those closest to us. Those who wanted to also drew theirs on the board. They all agreed the assignment made them aware of the people important in their lives. Some students insisted on putting in pets, who were, in many cases, just as close or closer to them than people. They also commented how they hadn't been so aware of how some people are closer to them than others. We found the people we have the most recent contact with are often included in the atom where they might have been left out or not placed so closely at another time.

As I put my own Atom on the board during the next group meeting, I noticed a change in myself that started somewhere in psychodrama. I am funny. I actually have a sense of humor again. Sometimes now I go overboard at work and joke about things that are serious to me, like the 7th graders not finishing assignments. One cover-up for another, but it is nice not to be *So* intense all the time. In my Atom my parents are not as close as I feel they are in my head. In my Atom I am surrounded with girlfriends. In my Atom I have more friends in general than I think possible at 2 a.m. But, of course, it is a problem figuring out where to put myself on the board, just as I had almost forgotten my name that first day. One of these times, I'll figure out who and where I am.

The next Friday we are talking about our earliest memories and how early memories affect our present lives. Bob, a school teacher on sabbatical, has a session. He was married ten years ago and has a hearing problem he believes is psychosomatic. It seems to be none of us escapes from the traumas of our parents. Some of us just deal with it better than others, but we all carry skeletons from our past. Bob is so tense and hurting. He has sharp stone features with fine bones, all pulled together above the nose and the tension in his whole body is never let out.

Suddenly I start to flash back. I am eight years old and my mother is pregnant. She has locked herself in the bedroom and my father is standing with me just outside the door. We don't know what to do. We both feel guilty that the woman on the other side feels bad. I do not know what exactly is the matter. I do not know how to make things better. I feel sick to my stomach. Vaguely I hear Bob talking about his father, and what a bully the father was. I see Bob stiff and tense on the stage, I see the little eight year old girl stiff and tense before the bedroom door. Someone is now saying, "Conflict, frustration and blockades are the mainstays of a session." I have a great fear of losing control of my fear and my feelings, so it all gets blocked up inside of me and transferred to hurting myself. It is easier to hurt myself than risk letting the feelings out. Poetry is also great therapy:

> You make me
> afraid of you
> cuz I'm small
> and not grown yet
> but I'll get big
> and hurt you for all the fear
> I have now.
> I won't let you
> throw me across the floor anymore
> or treat me like your pet goose
> you took out in back and . . .
> I'm five years old
> and I already know where to hide.
> I won't let you beat me
> with the ironing cord
> like you do mother

or dunk my head in cold water
every morning.
When I grow up
you'll be afraid of ME
for a change.

Judy has a session about her separation and upcoming divorce from her husband. That subject follows me everywhere. This week I saw *Scenes From A Marriage* by Bergman, and Michael, the one male I'll let close to me, is having to pick me up off the floor every other minute. It's like being married all over again. Now, in the psychodrama group it's like seeing the movie all over again. Will I never stop identifying????

There will be no continuation of these confessions to find out if I do become more objective. This is it. The ten psychodrama sessions I signed up for are over. I still have my hives, my weight is leaving more to be desired at every meal, I don't hate my mother anymore though because now I hate my brother (who is spoiled, but that's another story). So Psychodrama didn't give me an identity or make any miracle cures of me. But I did become more open and I did learn how universal my problems really are.

Psychodrama is a method that can range in impact from a simplistic attempt at solving immediate life problems on to a method that is not locked in by time, space, role, symbol, image, or philosophical meaning. In some measure, Susan's chronicle reflects this type of multidimensional effect. By entering into the more developed psychodramatic scenarios presented further on, you are urged to not simply respond to the clinical or therapeutic implications of the session, as important as this aspect of psychodrama is, but to also understand and participate in psychodrama in terms of its philosophical and dramaturgical qualities and impacts. Kian, "in pursuit of Paulette," not only presented an emotional problem but also dramatized a dimension of life that has meaning to many people.

The dramaturgical quality of psychodrama provides a complex of social scenes that have meaning on several levels for the protagonist, the group, and the larger society. Beyond its focus on therapy and problem-solving, psychodrama reveals the sometimes epic and peak experiences of life. No doubt the best way for you to experience psychodrama is to participate in a group session. Short of that, entering into the emotional spirit of the sessions that follow and responding to the scenarios' therapeutic insights and broader philosophical meaning can provide a valuable experience.

In summary, in order to maximize your personal-emotional benefit from reading the scenarios presented here, I would suggest that you participate in the psychodramas in the following ways:

1. Try to identify emotionally with the protagonist and the scenes presented as if you are part of the live audience at the psychodrama.
2. Try to comprehend the protagonist's basic problem and the best possible alternative solutions within the framework of the protagonist's total life situation. In this regard, attempt to place yourself in the same position as the protagonist in each session. In short, attempt to become his or her double.
3. The "mirror of life" effect is important. Does the session obliquely or directly relate to anyone close to you, or to yourself? When you finish absorbing a scenario, reflect on your personal identification with the protagonist and the specific meaning of the session to your *own* life. If possible, read the scenarios in tandem with someone close to you and, with this person, discuss the meaning and implications of the psychodrama for your own life.
4. Attempt to absorb the total meaning of the session in the most generalized and philosophical sense. For example, in relating to Kian's "in pursuit of Paulette," in what respects is your life in general a pursuit of past peak experiences? Consider Ralph's session: How did your parents discipline you? In terms of Phil and Selma's session: Did you or do you plan to marry for the same, or different reasons? Or, as another example, reflect on Helen's session with her dying mother. To what extent in American culture do we effectively relate to the meaning of death? How completely honest should we be or can we be with our loved ones? Does part of ourselves die with the death of a significant person in our life space?

The contemplation of these varied issues will enhance your participation in the scenarios presented and are offered as guides for most effectively participating in the psychodramatic process.

CHAPTER

2

Scenarios of Life

PSYCHODRAMA sessions tend to reflect and chronicle in an understandable microcosmic form the problems and conflicts that masses of people are experiencing in the macrocosm of the society. Psychodramatic scenarios are more significant and revealing than news reports of happenings because the sessions penetrate beneath the surface of human events. Psychodramas reveal the deeper emotional level of people's experiences.

People socialized in the same society, growing up with many common cultural experiences, tend to go through many parallel conflicts, dilemmas, and problems. Although no two sessions are ever the same, basic themes of our culture often emerge that are repeated in many sessions.

From the thousands of sessions I have directed or participated in, I have selected those scenarios that I feel reflect prototypical aspects of people's problems in our complex contemporary society. In the process of selection, I have also given priority to the inclusion of sessions that help delineate and explain the method of psychodrama.

Each scenario is presented in a somewhat different form. I have concluded that the simple verbatim presentation of actual transcripts of sessions often inadequately describe the emotion and meaning of the experience. The outstanding literary artist—a Tolstoy, a Faulkner, or a Shakespeare—presents only quintessential scenes and dialogue, giving adequate priority to the most important points and meaning of the overall story.

In a parallel way, to properly present a psychodrama, I find it is necessary to describe core scenes with nuances of dialogue, body positions, turning points of revelation, insights, the use of techniques, group moods, and the director's goals and therapeutic hypothesis in order to convey the real meaning of a session. In this presentation, therefore, some sessions will appear almost verbatim and others will be described using a minimum of actual dialogue. In all cases, I will use the descriptive form I consider most appropriate for illuminating each psychodramatic scenario's basic theme and meaning.

Fathers and Sons

A young, slender, shy man, neatly dressed, steps from the group. I ask him to introduce himself. (This self-presentation is important to almost every session in order to tune the group and the protagonist into the protagonist's self-concept.) "My name is Dan and I'm twenty-two. I work in an office as a clerk. I dropped out of college; it was just too hard for me. I'm alone. I would like to have a girlfriend but I'm too shy and unsure of myself. I don't think I'm man enough for most women."

L.Y.: Where do you live?
D.: I left home last year, against my parents' wishes.

We go to the scene when he leaves home. Auxiliary egos play his father and mother. It becomes apparent as the session unfolds that his basic conflict is with his domineering father, not his mother. We note that as he talks to his father in the session, he is overtly obedient, repeatedly saying, "Yes, sir," but on the body level, he clenches his fists so tightly his knuckles are white and almost breaking. His father storms around, essentially telling him in different ways, "You're a little baby. You can't make it in the world without my support. Therefore, you'll do exactly what I say." The young man is directed to reverse roles with his father. (This is done for two reasons: [1] To check whether the auxiliary ego is properly playing the role and [2] to check out the *son's perception* of his father's attitude toward him.) In the role of the father, the son continues to act belligerent and domineering. (This confirms that the auxiliary ego was close to the reality of the father, at least in the son's mind.)

L.Y.: You are now your dad. How old a man are you?
DAN AS FATHER: Fifty-four.
L.Y.: What's your name?
DAN AS FATHER: Dan.
L.Y.: No, you are now your father. What's your name?
DAN AS FATHER: Oh. Roy.
L.Y.: Does anyone in the group want to ask Roy here a question?
GROUP MEMBER: Do you love your son?
DAN AS ROY: I say I do, but I never show it. I don't know how. My father [Dan's grandfather] never showed me any affection either.
G.M.: Why don't you love your son?
DAN AS ROY: First of all, get one thing straight. I never wanted the little bastard. She [his wife] trapped me into this marriage by purposely getting knocked up. My son Dan's a puny little shit. I wanted my son to be an athlete, someone more aggressive. He's a sissy.

I now have Dan, who is visibly shaken by his pronouncements in the role of his father, return to his own role.

L.Y.: Okay, Dan. Here's your father. (The auxiliary ego returns as his father.) Tell him what you really think of him.
DAN (red-faced, almost sobbing): I can't. He's twice my size and he beats me. I'm scared of him.

The group and the director become aware of the disparity be-
tween Dan's perception of his father and reality. Dan is 6'3", but
he still perceives his father from a little boy's perspective.

L.Y.: I'm going to put in another Dan, as a double to help you
encounter your father.

The director selects a member of the group who is over six feet
and around two hundred pounds. He stands beside Dan. The
conversation continues with the father berating Dan and "little
Danny" as a "punk" and a "sissy." Dan and his double are con-
forming to type. The double emits exaggeratedly obedient "Yes,
sirs," which Dan, red-faced, repeats in subservience. His clenched
fists and body posture belie the obedient son he is overtly playing.
   Suddenly, after I give a direction to the double, the double
blurts out:
   "I hate your fuckin' guts. You son-of-a-bitch, I can't stand you
anymore—you're driving me nuts!!!"

As Dan's double blurts this out, Dan opens up and begins to
physically lunge at his father. Animal grunts and screams emerge
from his body. He holds onto his father's throat (psychodramatically, "the throat" is a rolled-up newspaper held in position by
the auxiliary ego playing the father) and groans in agony. These
groans of past repressed pain go on for several minutes—*without*
interference from the director. Dan has begun to feel his pain
and years of hostility toward his father that he has never expressed because of his fear and desire to be a "good boy."

I give the auxiliary ego a pillow to hold in front of him. And
Dan is told:

L.Y.: Okay, you can hit him.
DAN: I can't hit my father.
L.Y.: First of all, this is not really your father, so you can't hurt
"him." One thing we can do in psychodrama is determine the size
and shape of your hostility. You've been carrying these unexpressed
feelings around with you all your life. Now you have an opportunity to see where you're at. Just go with your feelings. All of us
here want to help you. The group expresses their involvement with
Dan and their desire to help.

At first Dan, with the support of his double, begins to viciously
punch the pillow (symbolically his father) and cry hysterically.
As he begins to act out physically, it's apparent he is enjoying

this expression of pent-up hatred. He begins to smile and says, "I really want to choke the bastard again."

He begins to choke the pillow still held by the auxiliary ego playing the role of his father.

Much of the anger has been expelled, and I attempt to focus the session from catharsis into insight.

L.Y.: Okay. Now I want you to punch the pillow as if it were your father. But with each punch, I want you to state why you're punching him.

The protagonist throws a hard punch with all of his might.

L.Y.: What's that for?

DAN: For never wanting me as your son!

Another punch.

L.Y.: What's that for?

DAN: For making fun of me when I was a kid and telling people I was a sissy.

Another punch.

L.Y.: What's that for?

DAN: For the times you got drunk and beat up my mother.

Dan is sobbing but under control as he now reviews methodically his reasons for hostility toward his father.

Another punch.

L.Y.: What's that for?

DAN: For being ashamed of me and not taking me anywhere.

This goes on, with several other deep complaints being brought to the surface. Now that the negative anger and hostility have been somewhat dispelled:

L.Y. to the auxiliary ego Father: Okay, hug your son.

DAN: I don't want him to do it.

L.Y.: Yes, you do. See what it feels like.

The father hugs his son, and Dan breaks into tears in his "father's" arms.

DAN: Dad, that's what I always wanted from you—just for you to love me and tell me I'm okay.

FATHER: I've always loved you, son, but I never learned how to express it. Can you forgive me?

DAN: I don't know.

L.Y. and Group: Why don't you forgive him?

DAN: I'll try, but I'm not sure I can do it.

L.Y.: If you can really forgive him, you'll also give up that ball of hostility in your gut that you have from hating him. You will free yourself from being entrapped by your anger. You accept the self-doubt and low self-concept generated by your father. He has, because of his own needs, carried on a propaganda campaign against you all your life. He had defined you as a punk, rejected kid and you believe these negative things about yourself. It's true you were rejected, but we here see you as a fine person who has been victimized by an oppressive father.

At this point, Dan (as is usually true of a protagonist) is exhausted. The director sits down with him in front of the group.
L.Y. (to group): Dan has courageously given of himself to the group. Now is the time to hear your points of identification and empathy with his session. Remember, this is not the time for the analysis of Dan's psychodynamics. We'll get to that later. This is the time to share your personal identification with Dan and the group.

At this point, different members of the group share by expressing their thoughts and feelings about their fathers; and in several cases, women indicate that the same pattern obtained with their mothers. Following are summarized some typical reactions. This was done by having members of the group come on stage and talk to an auxiliary ego as their father or mother, or in some cases simply soliloquize their feelings. Some sons and daughters were more vehement than others.
CAROL: My hostility toward my mother was kicked up by Dan's session. She was an alcoholic and she took care of me in cycles. There were times when she was an affectionate, caring mother. Then I would be abandoned for days, sometimes weeks, when she was on a bender. Maybe I would have been better off if I had never seen her as a good mother, because it made the pain of the bad days worse.

She was defeated by life and she tried to plant that attitude in me. Her favorite expressions were "What's the use" and "You can't win no matter how hard you try." I know now that an early age she programmed me for defeat.

I became really mad at her when I was a teenager, and I saw other mothers who took care of their daughters. You know, mothers who fixed their daughters' hair and went shopping with them. By comparison, I realized I was shortchanged. I felt alone and rejected. Most of the time I had no mother to guide me, and I was rejected by the other kids. This fed and built up in me a sense of being a nobody. Rejection meant there was something terribly wrong with me.

I hated my mother for all of these feelings, because I always felt she was responsible for my pain—and she was. I now understand she had her own problems, but a little kid doesn't understand that. All she understands from rejection is that there's something terribly wrong with her. For a long time I escaped into drugs, to kill my pain. Now I'm beginning to understand what happened to me, and I feel better about myself. But seeing Dan being oppressed by his father reminded me of my own scene.

SARAH: I identified with Dan in regard to his father's rejection. My mother was more subtle. She always acted "as if" she loved me. But she only loved me if I did *exactly* what she wanted. I had to suppress the real me. She was and is a total show-off. Everything she ever did was for effect. The house was always spotless and she had my room all in white. To her I was not a person but another ornament that she showed off like the furniture. She cut my hair a special way—*that she liked*. I dressed the way she liked. To her I was an inanimate object. Carol shouldn't feel too bad about being left alone. Although it looked like I was cared for, there was no concern for me as a person. I was like an extension of her ego needs and image.

She's still after me, even though I'm twenty-five. She wants me to marry someone *she* can show off. Someone that will make her look good. She doesn't care who I like, and I'm still battling with her.

I've often wished she was dead. I've dreamed about killing her. I really identified with Dan choking his father. I want a session sometime where I can do my mother in.

Several young men in the group come on stage to express their feelings toward their fathers, with an auxiliary ego assuming the necessary father role.

ERIC: Like Dan's father, you never were there for me either. You never loved me. You never did anything with me. Never took me fishing, never played ball, never once took me to a ball game. Always sitting in front of the goddamned television, reading the papers, or going to work.

BILL: No matter what I did, it was never good enough. When I told you I came in second in a race at school, it was always, "Why didn't you come in first?" If I told you I got an A in math, you'd say "But you only got a B+ in English." I could never do anything to please you. I never got any approval from you for anything and I tried so hard and *dammit* (as if angry with himself) I'm still trying.

JERRY: I thought my problem was with my mother, but it was with you, you son-of-a-bitch. You let her take over. Why did you let her talk to you that way? Why did you let her push you around? Why weren't you a man so that I could learn to be a man? I'm ashamed to have you as a father, you're so weak. How could you take her constant nagging and harassing without getting mad?

Another group member, Todd, appears warmed up to a "mini-session," a session revolving around one issue. With auxiliaries I set the scene for Todd in which mother is belittling father to trigger his pain and give Todd the opportunity to "violently" act out his pent-up frustration, anger, and pain. At this point, a pillow either held or placed on the floor, or a battoca (the cushion-like weapon used in group sessions to express anger) is placed in the protagonist's hands over a table on which he could pound out his rage. The protagonist seizes the battoca and exclaims as he furiously beats the table.

TODD: I was just a little kid. Why did you have to beat me up all the time? I never even did anything wrong. And you used to hit my mother, too, for no good reason. You were always drunk and mean, and if it wasn't for my mom we wouldn't even have had food in the house. I hate you, but how can I hate a dead person? I was just marking time until I was old enough and big enough to beat the shit out of you like you did us, and then you died—you bastard (breaks into tears).

Another member of the group, John, signals for recognition and is warmed up to "talk to" his father.

JOHN: I'm not sure how I feel about you. I know I always had to tiptoe around the house so as not to disturb you, and I always had to be very careful not to say anything that would upset you.
L.Y.: Are you angry with him?
JOHN: I guess I am but I can't tell him. I feel too guilty.
L.Y.: Now is your chance to tell him your true feelings without hurting him, since he's not in reality here.
JOHN: How can I be angry with him when I feel sorry for him? He's a sick man who's been beridden for as long as I can remember. How can I say anything mean or angry to a man who's sick with a heart condition? He'd always scream at my mother to bring him this and bring him that and then berate her. He'd attack us personally, tell us we were ugly and no good. He was full of bitterness and took it out on us. But my mom always apologized for him and

told us if we said one word against him we'd be sorry, because upsetting him might shorten his life. I can't hit him or yell at him even here, now, I feel too guilty, too sorry for him, or at least that's the trip my mother laid on me. Everything revolved around "poor Daddy."

The first protagonist, Dan, obviously kicked off many negative feelings of others in the group toward their fathers and mothers. There were, of course, a number of people in the group who indicated that their parents were caring and loving. They felt no problem with their parents; their difficulty stemmed from other issues. I pointed out to the group that at least in this session we were focused on negative relationships. (We often have a session that shows a positive prototype of the negative interpersonal relationship someone is experiencing.) Most of the others who felt parental problems were put "on hold" for future sessions, although several felt a degree of insight and catharsis through Dan's session.

Dan said he felt better knowing that there were other people who had experienced his life situation. Before we ended the session, Dan felt forgiving and acted out a scene where he symbolically forgave his father for all of the negative things Dan felt he had experienced from him.

At this point in the session, the group was prepared for some more generalized analysis of the session, and I delineated several general points.

Dan went through four typical phases that appear in many sessions when a "child," male or female, breaks through into expressing his grievances and the pain he has felt because he found it necessary to suppress his real feelings:

Phase I—The recognition of the size and shape of his hostility.
Phase II—Cathartic acting-out of hostility toward parental object of pain.
Phase III—Expression of primal pain (nonverbal groans and crying) that in a sense mourns the felt absence of desired parental love.
Phase IV—Forgiveness and possible expression of love.

In Phase I the protagonist locates and recognizes his enormous pent-up hostility about long-term grievances. The group and the psychodrama director, through a double, often find it necessary to explicate the protagonist's grievance.

Following this (in Phase II), the protagonist should be given the opportunity to specifically express his rage for the many years of pain. The protagonist, by punching a pillow, using a battoca, kicking, or whatever form his venom takes, will typically express his hostility in a torrent of anger. Curiously, everyone seems to harbor his own peculiar pattern of expressing his anger. For most, the pillow or battoca is fine, but some people want to use poison, a gun, or other forms of destruction.

In this phase of expression, it is important to have the protagonist express his explicit grievances. As Dan said, with each punch, "This is for not wanting me. . . . This is for never approving of anything I did. . . ," etc. This process helps the protagonist to more clearly understand the inadequacies that have been projected onto him and the degree to which he has accepted this propaganda, which usually results in self-hatred and a low self-concept.

At this point, Phase III, the protagonist begins to feel his deeper pain and typically cry and groan with deep emotion. It is important to let the protagonist "feel" his pain and not cut off his expression prematurely by soothing him. It is necessary for the protagonist to take whatever time is required to experience his emotions in this context with the parent (auxiliary ego) present.

Phase IV, the expression of love and forgiveness, does not usually emerge in most sessions as readily as the earlier expression of hostility. My experience reveals that this phase of forgiveness and affection can seldom be fully expressed (except superficially) *until* the protagonist has *first* fully expressed his feelings of hostility. Once this has happened, however, the protagonist is in a position to forgive and try to forget. As the director, I always emphasize that the symbolic and sometimes real expression of forgiveness is not for the benefit of the object-parent but is a beneficial relief for the protagonist. When they can forgive, they divest themselves of the necessity of carrying around their rage and maintaining a vendetta that more often than not impairs the protagonist's happiness and produces self-defeating behavioral patterns.

Occasionally, a protagonist can experience these four phases in one session. It is more likely, however, that the full experience will take place through a number of psychodramatic experiences (which may be combined with individual therapeutic sessions). It is usually necessary to be the central protagonist in at least one session in order to go through this pattern of self-liberation; however, it should be emphasized that people can achieve some (or even all) facets of this experience by deep involvement in sessions with other protagonists who are going through this process. A person, therefore, can benefit from psychodrama not only from the position of protagonist but from being an actively involved group member.

The Seven-Year Twitch

Many psychodrama sessions revolve around the complex joy and pain of being married or the relationship of "living together." The psychodramatist is neutral about attempting to keep a couple married or together. There is no moral dictum imposed on the situation implying that marriage—or a relationship—is "good" or "bad." Emphasis is placed on the function and happiness that the relationship produces.

A major goal of a session is to help the participants determine for themselves the best course of action (continuance or separation) based on the evidence that emerges during the psychodramatic exploration of the marital condition.

L.Y.: Who here has a problem they would like to present?

A young man of around twenty-five talks briefly about his

arguments with his wife over the handling of their children. He wants more discipline, and she is more laissez-faire.

L.Y.: Okay, we might go with that. Let's hear from someone else.
A young woman says, "I've been separated from my husband for almost a year and my divorce becomes final in a month."
L.Y.: How do you feel about it?
Y.W.: Just wonderful.
L.Y.: Well, if you feel that way, there's really not much point in exploring your divorce. Psychodrama is most effective as a vehicle for probing and assessing relationships that are problematic.

At this point, another young lady in the group named Jane begins to talk.

JANE: I'm trying to separate from my husband, and I'm in great pain about it. I don't know how he can be so calm about being separated. Coming to a decision on what I really want to do is driving me nuts!
L.Y.: You seem quite warmed up to your problem. How does the group feel about moving ahead with Jane?

The group assents, with several people saying that they have similar problems or have been "through it."

L.Y.: Okay. Come on up, Jane. First introduce yourself to the group.
JANE: I'm twenty-eight and I've been married to Bill for seven years. I've never been with another man sexually. Bill is like the only family I've known. But I'm just bored to death with him!
L.Y.: Let's get into the role-playing. When you talk too much about a problem, it dissipates the act-hunger. Have you told him about your feelings?
JANE: That's part of the problem. He doesn't listen. He's like a stone.
L.Y.: Okay. When was the last time you confronted him?
JANE: He just came back from two days on a boating trip. He went alone with another guy. We had agreed to separate briefly.
L.Y.: Is there someone here who looks like Bill who could play him?
JANE: Well, no one in particular.
L.Y.: Okay. Can this be Bill? (I select a young man from the group.)
JANE: Yeah. He even looks a little like him.

L.Y.: Okay, set up the scene. Where are you? Where is he? What does the room look like? It's important for you and the group to move into the ambience of the situation.

Jane sets up the scene in their bedroom. There's a water bed and very little furniture. It's midnight and he's just returned from a trip.

BILL: Boy, am I tired.

JANE: Bill, I have to talk to you.

BILL: Oh, Christ. Let's not do that number again. I'm tired.

JANE (*pleading*): Please, Bill. Just listen to me, I *hurt!*

BILL: That's not my fault.

JANE: Don't you know I'm going to leave you—if you don't talk to me. There's no communication.

BILL: Save that communication bullshit for your sociology class. I don't feel we have any problem. I'm very happy.

JANE: I'm miserable. Can't you see it? I'm twenty-eight and my goddamn eye twitches!

BILL: It's not my fault.

JANE: Nothing is! Please listen to me. You know I read books, I go to a class and hear new ideas. It turns me on. I come home and want to talk to you about the things that are important to me. . . .

BILL: I don't want to hear that shit! It's twelve o'clock. I've had a long trip. (*Pause*) Come on. Why don't we make love. (*He approaches her.*)

JANE: No, please don't do that to me. I don't feel like it. I want to talk.

BILL: Come on. Making love is communication. Come on. Everything will be fine.

JANE: Please don't. I'm not going to *submit* to you again.

At this point, I ask Jane if the auxiliary ego "Bill" has given an accurate portrayal. She says "pretty close." I then have her reverse roles. She becomes Bill and the auxiliary ego becomes "Jane." The action continues for a few minutes in the same vein.

L.Y.: Hold it a minute, Bill. (*Jane is now Bill.*) We're going to ask you a few questions (*to get her more into the role of Bill*). Tell us something about yourself. (The following dialogue is her response to me and questions from other members of the group.)

JANE AS BILL: I'm thirty. I teach high school. I love my wife. And I don't know what's happened to her. She used to be quiet and cuddly, and she did the housework without any complaints. She was my little Janey. Now she runs to these classes. I think she even has another guy she's interested in. She wants to talk about a lot of bullshit I'm not interested in. She's changing and I'm the same. I don't know what she wants from me.

JANE (*played by the auxiliary ego*): I want you to understand. You bore me to death.

JANE AS BILL: I bore you. Who feeds you and takes care of you when you're sick and has supported you for seven goddamn years?

L.Y.: Okay, reverse roles.

Jane becomes herself again, and as the conversation continues in the same vein, I have the auxiliary ego who is playing Bill spread his arms in crucifixion style to reveal his "saintliness." "How can you do this to me? I've been so good. I've always been the kind of husband I promised you I would be when we got married."

JANE (*smiles*): God, he lays guilt on top of guilt on me. He's right. He has been so good. He's perfect. I feel like a complete bitch. But he bores me every way possible. In bed. In conversation. Everywhere. I want out. I'm suffocating.

L.Y.: How about your parents?

JANE: Oh, I knew that was coming.

We move into a scene with her mother and father. With them she plays little girl Janey. She distorts the real situation to her parents and implies to them that Bill also wants out. We put in a double behind Jane who introduces the reality that she is the dissident. Jane tries to stifle her double when she blurts out the truth of her unilateral desire to leave Bill—she wants to hide this from her parents.

MOTHER: You get right home. You're a spoiled child. You'll never get a boy as wonderful as Bill. I'll fix it up. I'll call him.

JANE: No, Mother, please. I want to leave him.

FATHER (*to wife*): Tell your daughter to go right back to him. He's a wonderful boy. How can she even think of leaving him? It's your fault. You never raised her to be a real woman; a real woman takes care of the house, has babies.

JANE'S DOUBLE: Oh, God. Now I know why I'm so stuck. If I leave Bill, I'm not only leaving him, I'm leaving my mother and father. It scares me to death. These three people *are* my family. *I can't leave my only family.*

JANE: Yes, that's exactly right. There's something else I just realized. If I leave Bill, I have to give up the role of cute little Janey, the role I play with Bill and my mom and dad. It scares me. My identity as a grown woman isn't that secure.

BILL: If you leave me, you'll really be sorry. I'm so good to you.

JANE: Oh, fuck you, man. I can't stand you anymore. All you do is make me feel guilty about how *good* you are. I have to go.

L.Y. (*joking*): Now, now, "Little Janey" doesn't say "fuck you!"
In the next scene, I have Jane go back in time to her marriage ceremony. As she stands next to Bill in the church and the minister pronounces them man and wife, Jane soliloquizes:

JANE: Boy, am I lucky to get him. Little, fat, ugly me finally has a man! I'm not wild about him, but he's solid and right and my folks like him. In fact, they like him better than I do.
We next do a scene in an efficient divorce lawyer's office. He opens by detailing her rights and asks her to sign the final papers. As this goes on, Jane and her double soliloquize in debate:

JANE: I can't do this to him and my mom and dad. I feel like I'm betraying them.

JANE'S DOUBLE: I have to. It's my only chance to really be myself, instead of what they think they want. I'm tired of living up to their expectations.

JANE: That's right. It's now or never. When I married him I was ootzy-kootsie Janie. I've lost weight and I'm attractive. I'm tired of playing that childlike role for my husband and family. It demeans me. (To lawyer): Give me that divorce paper. I'll sign it.

Post-Discussion Responses—"The Family Court"

In some respects, the session and the post-discussion are like a nonlegal "family court" with the marriage on trial. I always have the auxiliary ego husband (especially if the real husband is not present) forcefully present his viewpoint. In terms of the judicial model, members of the group naturally emerge as "prosecutors" and defense witnesses in a dialectical debate on the marriage.

I have Jane and the various participants sit with me in a semi-circle in front of the group:

L.Y.: I want to ask Jack here (the man who played Bill) how he felt in the role. Very often the auxiliary ego picks up nuances of emotion that elude the director and the group.

JACK: Well, this session was really a mind-blower because I am Bill! My wife and I are going through the very same thing right now. We've even been married seven years. Except instead of my escaping up a river on a boat like Bill, I sublimate by riding horses. My wife says some of the same things to me that Jane was saying to Bill. I wasn't just playing Bill, *I was Bill*. I was really responding as myself to all kinds of demands being made on me that she never made before. Just because she's changed or grown or whatever, suddenly I'm not good enough as I am. I was fine for seven years, but now I'm not because she thinks she's changed. I feel stubborn about it, like she wants me to be somebody I'm not. I've never been a talkative person and I'm not openly demonstrative. My wife and I conflict in a lot of ways. I'm into science and she's into mysticism with all her new weird friends, and I'm not interested.

L.Y.: Let's hear from the rest of the group. First I want everyone here to be Bill and speak from his point of view. Even though he's not here, he has a right to be heard.

GROUP MEMBER 1 AS BILL (*inflaming her guilt*): Well, Jane, I just want you to know that even though I have been a devoted and loyal husband, have supported you, taken care of you when you've been ill, tried to cheer you when you've been down, and have loved you dearly, if you want to leave, it's your decision. I won't try to stop you.

G.M. 2 AS BILL (*begging*): Jane, I love you, please don't leave me. I'll do anything you ask. I'll even go for help with you even though it seems to go against my nature. I'll try to be more communicative and open, and I promise we'll find more things to do together. I'll listen to you and try to become interested in your work, but please don't leave me.

G.M. 3 AS BILL: You're acting very childish, Jane. All marriages have ups and downs. Don't do anything rash that you'll regret. I know we'll get through this and in time things will be back to the way they were.

L.Y.: Now in our post-discussion, let's hear from those members of the group who identified with Jane. Remember, no analysis at this time. Let's hear about your personal points of identification with Jane.

MARY: Well, I can really identify with you, not only with regard to your husband but to the whole family situation. My husband was the first guy I was ever really with. My parents were crazy about him and everything was neat until I started going back to school. Then I started discovering that *I* could be interesting, that *I* could attract friends on my own and hold my own in conversation. When this happened, he became very possessive and began trying to keep me down. I knew after a while that I could never go back to being the person I was and that he wasn't going to change.

My folks were living in Hawaii at the time, and they were very supportive for a while. They wrote these cheerful letters saying, "Okay, this is just a bad time for the two of you and we love you both, and know you'll work through this, we're counting on you," etc. When I finally made the decision to leave him and wrote them that I had left, I did not hear from them for a whole year (Mary begins to sob).

I was totally alone and scared to death, but I survived and I never knew how strong I could be. If I would have stayed in that situation with my husband, something in me would have died. I'm not saying everything is wonderful now. I get lonely living by myself and I sometimes miss having a man of my own, but I'm free and I'm finding out some very exciting things about who I am and what I can do. I'm sure it's just a matter of time before I meet a guy who's into learning and growing and who's secure enough to let me be who I am without trying to stifle me or push me into some kind of mold that he has set for me.

ALICE: I was married for eleven years, I have two children, and talk about guilt, I thought I was going to have a nervous breakdown. Like your husband, mine was, quote, "a good man." He always provided for us, he was dependable, he was a good father, he was a loyal husband—and he bored me to death. It got so bad that I not only couldn't go to bed with him but even having him touch me or kiss me was repugnant. For four years I lived in hell. I felt so damned sorry for him and so guilty. I became convinced that I was just a dissatisfied, no-good bitch.

My mother would always extoll his virtues and tell me that there's no better man, no better husband or father on this earth. If it wasn't for the children I would have left long before I did, but I kept thinking of how selfish I was to even think of depriving them of a father.

You're lucky, you don't have children. It makes it very difficult. What finally happened was that it became so intolerable that my girls were actually suffering from the situation and I felt that getting out would be healthier. We agreed to a trial separation, and I tell you that getting away from him was such a relief I felt as though I had been in prison for eleven years. I am happy right now; in fact, I can't ever remember being this happy in my entire life.

BETTE: Well, what happened with my husband and me is really kinda different from the experiences described so far. We started going together in high school and were married right after he graduated. It's funny, like Jane, I think we were together around seven years when I started getting very restless and feeling that I had missed out on a lot of fun by marrying so young. I felt it more intensely after I joined a woman's consciousness-raising group and began to compare my experiences with the experiences of other women.

I mean, Bob was one of the first guys I dated, I was a virgin when we met, and I never had the adventure of having dates with different guys. Also, I went right from the world of living with my parents to living with him and had never been on my own. Anyway, after around seven years, I just felt that if I didn't break away and try making it on my own that I'd be trapped forever. So we agreed on a trial separation, and it was really rough at first.

I felt like a little girl, kind of helpless and frightened. Also, I wasn't prepared for the solitude of living alone. Actually, after the first month, I wanted to go back, but I knew my motivation at that time was to find security, not just that I loved him and wanted to be with him. So I dated and I found a job I liked. I met a lot of people and I felt that it was very good for me.

But I also realized after several short-term lousy relationships that Bob was really the man I wanted as my husband, and fortunately it wasn't too late. We have a little girl now, and he understands that I've got to feel free to work or go to school or whatever, and we're very happy. I guess all I wanted at the seven-year point was a little adventure.

Jane was now better armed for her decision, not only by the revelations of her session but by the feedback of experience provided by other members of the group. Although she made a decision for divorce in the session, it did not fully carry over into the reality of her life. The session did, however, enrich her understanding of the possible consequences of the several alternatives open to her. I gave her the *psychodramatic prescription* of going home and relating the total session to him. Even though he was not present at the session when she told him in great detail about the scenario of their marriage from her viewpoint, it had a carom-shot impact. They began to work harder at communicating, and in subsequent sessions it appeared that they had made progress.

Role-Playing Sexual Fantasies

Almost everyone has had sexual fantasies, but very few people have acted them out in life. In some cases, the enactment would land the protagonist in court and possibly prison. Not so in psychodrama. Many people have acted-out modified versions of their fantasy. (The actual sexual act is not permitted, even in psychodrama.) It is, however, a therapeutic possibility that may be experimentally tried in the future. The positive result of many of these sessions is that the protagonist becomes more aware of the nature of the fantasy and the fact that other people have these or similar fantasies. In some cases, when a fantasy was acted out in the presence of a spouse, it was later enacted in life. In the psychodrama of a sexual fantasy, people learn that they are not alone, and the concern of many that they are "crazy" because of their peculiar fantasies is ameliorated. Also, in most cases, acting-out in psychodrama tends to reveal something about the psychodynamic base of the fantasy.

In one memorable session in this genre, a protagonist came forward and presented her husband's sexual ritual and her apparent retaliatory fantasy.

L.Y.: Set up the situation.
   She is in bed with her husband.
MARLENE: I'm subjected to this ritual almost every morning.
L.Y.: Reverse roles. Be your husband.
MARLENE AS JOHN: I'm masturbating. (*She feigns masturbation.*) Oh, I'm about to come. Oh, Marlene, come here!
   As John, she partially mounts the auxiliary who plays her.
MARLENE AS JOHN (*apparently relieved*): Boy, that was great. Okay, now quick get the "Start."
L.Y.: What's "Start"?

MARLENE: It's an instant orange drink. They advertise by saying, "Once you drink 'Start' you can't stop." (*group laughs*).
L.Y.: Reverse roles.
MARLENE: I run and mix him a big glass of "Start," which he gulps down. He's off to work and I'm left behind totally sexually frustrated most of the time. It's only once in a great while that he makes reasonable love to me. Most of the time he masturbates. I get on him for a minute or less. Then I get the "Start."
L.Y.: So that's the ritual. Now let's see the fantasy you mentioned.
MARLENE: It happens in my dreams. I have this one recurring dream I've had around twenty times.
L.Y.: Okay, you're dreaming—but enact your dream. Stand up. Where are you? Just soliloquize.
MARLENE: I'm in the woods. Ah! There's one. What a big magnificent bear (she points to a big, handsome man in the group who spontaneously assumes the role of a bear).
BEAR: You want me?
MARLENE: Oh, yes I do. Come over here, you big, beautiful stud.
BEAR: Sure. Anything you say.
MARLENE: Now look at me. Your prick is absolutely enormous. Wow, come here now. I'm going to train you to do it to me exactly as I like it.
She draws bear close to her.
MARLENE: Come on, Mr. Bear, fuck me!
(Auxiliary ego bear looks at L.Y. questioningly.)
L.Y.: Obviously we can't physically act this out. Just embrace her.
MARLENE: Okay. That's it! Now slow down. Okay, get down. You have a marvelous tongue. That's it. Beautiful.
L.Y.: Is that it?
MARLENE: Yes, more or less. Except in my fantasy I have around five bears, and they are all perfectly trained to make love to me exactly the way I want it. Do you think I'm nuts?

It was obvious that Marlene's relationship with her husband and her subservience to his needs required more intensive analysis and therapeutic attention. However, the group concluded, in the context of this limited enactment, that Marlene's fantasy was a retaliatory expression. As one group member expressed it: "Your fantasy is a reaction-formation. With your husband, you have no control over him. You just service his ridiculous selfish needs and you're frustrated. With the bears, you're at the opposite extreme.

You train them to do exactly as you like, and they fully satisfy you."

In a further discussion of Marlene's fantasy with the group, several women revealed that they too fantasized having sex with animals. Marlene seemed relieved that she was not alone, and in future sessions we worked on her peculiar relationship with her husband.

In another session provoked by Marlene, another lady in the group detailed her consistent dreamlike fantasy. In it she invariably found herself in a corral. Everyone in the corral is a stud bull and she's the only cow. In the session, we had several men play bulls who surrounded her and wanted her. She thoroughly enjoyed the expression of her fantasy and exclaimed at one point: "Oh, my God. Isn't it wonderful. All of these luscious big bulls want me!" The interpretation of the group was that the protagonist wanted more male attention and that her fantasy involved achieving super-attention from men. This fantasy, also, obviously opened up sessions around the lady's more complex life situation.

In another session, a woman enacted a very *precise* fantasy that revolved around a recurrent dream. A man would pick her up on a date, romance her, then drive out to the country. He would then become gently domineering.

MAN (*played by protagonist*): Okay. Now get out of the car. Get over there in front of the car headlights. Okay, take off all your clothes. Now I'm going to make wild, passionate love to you.

In her dream, the man would come to the front of the car and make love to her in the glare of the headlights, almost as if they were on stage. She revealed that she often fantasized that this was happening when she made love to her husband to heighten her feeling, and she also conjured up the dream when she was masturbating.

In the session, we arrived at no precise interpretation of why she desired to be sexually "in the spotlight," but she claimed to feel better after psychodramatically acting it out. This response appeared to be the general consensus after the enactment of a fantasy. It made people feel better to know that others shared sexual fantasies or had their own.

A common "revelation" in sexual psychodramas was the fact that during the sex act people fantasized other people (sometimes movie stars) or erotic scenes. The group's consensual responses seemed to be valuable in relieving disconcerting feelings in the protagonist of feeling "guilty," "strange," or "crazy." In many post-psychodrama group discussions, a conclusion reached was that basically people are not monogamous and sexual excitation often related to people other than one's spouse. Most people felt that excessive acting-out of drives for others would disrupt their functional monogamous relationship. Consequently, they concluded that fantasizing other people or scenes in the sex act was a natural, effective, and perhaps necessary adjustment to the maintenance of monogamy. Talking out these issues was not as useful or graphic as acting them out with a group. These mini-psychodramas, in a group setting, appeared to give all of its members some insights into their fantasies and the underlying reasons for having them.

Preventing a Murder?

When I worked with violent gangs in New York, I was often confronted with emergency problems that required immediate attention.* The potential problem often involved violence, and on several occasions I was able to head off potentially violent consequences with a preventive psychodrama.

In one case, a gang leader that I knew, accompanied by two friends, accosted me as I was walking down the street, pulled out a switchblade knife, and announced that he was on his way to kill a member of another gang from a nearby neighborhood on the Upper West Side of Manhattan.

* For a more detailed analysis, see Lewis Yablonsky, *The Violent Gang* (New York: Macmillan, 1962, Penguin, 1966).

I was somewhat prepared in advance for this emergency possibility, since on a continuing basis I had made sociometric tests that revealed the relationships of various gangs and gang networks in the area. I knew the gangs that were feuding and the leadership patterns of each group. More than that, I had run psychodrama sessions with many gang members, including the youths in my presence. I invited the trio to my office to talk it over.

They agreed to go along with me, and on the way I of course considered the question: Why did the youth stop me before he went to stab his intended victim? I suspected the chances were good that he really did not want to commit this violence and wanted me to help him find a way out.

The "Ape," as this boy was called by the gang, was openly defiant and upset. His opening remark was: "Man, I'm packin'; I got my blade [switchblade knife] right here. I'm going to cut the shit out of those mother-fuckin' Dragons [the rival gang]. I'm goin' up and get them now . . . once and for all." Briefly, he had his knife and was going to stab any Dragon gang boy he met that day.

After some brief conversation in my office, the boys agreed to get into a psychodrama session.

The session began with the use of one of the gang boys as an auxiliary ego in the role of the potential victim. A paper ruler replaced the knife (for obvious reasons), and the "killing" was acted-out in my office under controlled psychodramatic conditions.

The psychodrama had all of the elements of a real gang killing. The Ape (as protagonist) cursed, fumed, threatened, and shouted at the victim, who hurled threats and insults in return. Ape worked himself into a frenzy and then stabbed the auxiliary ego victim with the paper knife. The psychodramatic victim fell dead on the floor.

The Ape was then confronted with the consequences of his act in all of its dimensions, including the effect on his family. He began to regret what he had done and was particularly remorseful when (psychodramatically) an auxiliary ego playing the role of a court judge sentenced him "to death in the electric chair." In order to reinforce the meaning of the consequences of his potential act, I had him reverse roles and, from the position of the judge, *he* sentenced *himself* to death. This performance had a profound emotional impact on the Ape.

The psychodrama accomplished at least two things for this very potential killer: (1) He seemed less motivated to kill, since he had already completed the act psychodramatically. (2) He was confronted with the consequences of his rash act; this was an added dimension of consideration. Most violence-prone people are unable to think ahead in a situation to the outcome.

These factors possibly served as a deterrent to the actual commission of a murder. Of course, this boy required and received other sessions, which sought to deal with his more basic personality problems. Moreover, considerably more work was attempted on the gang networks, so as to minimize their potential for violence. However, the emergency psychodrama, *in situ,* did deter the possibility of Ape committing a homicide, at least on that particular day.

Escape

Violence is often turned on oneself in peculiar ways. Most people are aware of the dire self-destructive consequences of alcoholism and drug addiction. Despite this awareness of the self-destructive consequences of using drugs or alcohol to excess, many people encounter forces that propel them into lives of self-destruction. It is these underlying forces that produce the symptoms of drug abuse.

A psychodrama session I ran with an attractive young lady in a group of heroin addicts was most revealing about her motivation to addiction. Her escape through drugs has broader implications for revealing the manner in which others become addicted to drugs and alcohol. The protagonist, Diana, was twenty at the time of the session and had been a heroin addict for four years.

Diana, the group, and I agreed that the psychodrama session could productively focus on the causal factors, the sequence of events, that led to her first fix of heroin.

The session was taped. Because of the coherence of the session and the protagonist's articulateness, this session is best presented dominantly with the original dialogue of the session.

Diana is motivated to resolve her problem, and steps up on the psychodrama stage.

L.Y.: What are your first recollections as a child of trouble in your life?

DIANA: Of trouble? Oh. I have a lot of it. Oh, wow. I had so many problems . . . I remember once when I was like three, watching my father beat up my mother. And I saw blood shoot out her nose. (*With both forefingers she traces a trajectory from her nostrils outward.*) All over the walls. I was sitting on the sofa with my legs up, you know, like this. (*She demonstrates the position.*) And I couldn't stop screaming. That's just one flash that I have.

L.Y.: You're three years old. Here is your mother and father. (*Auxiliary egos step forward.*) Be there, almost as if in a dream, like right here. There's no sound emitting from you. Maybe muffled cries. I want you to double with her. Your parents are beating the hell out of each other, and you're sitting there watching.

The double takes her position behind Diana. Two "parents" (auxiliary egos) start their action of simulating the beating.

DIANA (*staring at them for a while before recollecting*): . . . They're drunk. And she's calling him names. I'm watching and I'm . . .

As she watches the beating, she suddenly emits a loud and prolonged scream of terror. The screaming goes on for several minutes and she almost seems unable to stop. As she screams, the auxiliary ego father and mother simulate beating on each other.

L.Y.: What are you thinking? I know that you're only three years old, but in psychodrama we can have three-year-olds express their feelings.

DIANA: I don't know. I'm terrified. Oh! I'm terrified. I don't know what's happening . . .

L.Y.: What else are you thinking?

DIANA: I want them to stop . . . I don't want to look. . . .

DIANA'S DOUBLE: I don't know what to do. I don't know where to go.

DIANA: I want to call for my mother.

L.Y.: Do you call her?

DIANA: No, I don't. I can't do it. I can't stop screaming. That's all I can do, scream and cry.

(When a person is as quickly and intensely in touch with her feelings as Diana was, there is no point in prolonging the emotion.)

L.Y.: Don't scream again. I want you to try to intellectualize your feelings. What do you think as you look at your mother being hit? What occurs to you?

DIANA: I don't know what they are doing. I just see that something terrible is happening. Blood is coming out of my mother's nose. They act like they are killing each other.

DIANA'S DOUBLE: I am so scared . . . so scared . . .

DIANA: I am really scared. I wish they'd stop.

L.Y.: You want to get out of here.

DIANA: I don't know what I want to do. All I can do is sit and scream. That's all I can do. I can't move. I can't get away. I can't do anything.

L.Y.: At three years old, you really don't have adequate words to express your feelings. But right now, Diana, you do have words. And I want you to tell your mother how you feel about her.

DIANA: Is something wrong with you? I know that when you drink certain things happen. You don't walk straight. And your breath smells of liquor. I don't trust you. I think you are going to drop me when you pick me up, that you are going to hurt me. When we drive in the car, we slam into things and you slam your fingers in the car door. I'm afraid of you when you are drunk.

L.Y.: Okay, Diana, you are now around six years old. Did you ever get a chance to tell her what you think of her?

DIANA: No. I don't want to hurt her feelings.

L.Y.: Don't worry now about hurting her feelings, since this, obviously, really isn't your mother. In psychodrama we can say anything we want.

DIANA: I wish you wouldn't try to kiss me because you make me sick. You take a drink of my milk sometimes, and you take a bit of my food, and I feel repelled by you. You've got food running down . . . (she touches her face, simulating the food running down her neck) . . . in front of your dress. You smell like liquor and you're sloppy.

"MOTHER": It's all right . . . it's all right, baby. Come on, give Mama a kiss.

DIANA'S DOUBLE: You always scare me. You always scare me.

Diana looks at the mother attentively. An expression of disgust builds up on her face.

"MOTHER": It's all right. It's all right, baby. Everything is okay. Everything will be all right. Come on, give me a kiss, goddamn it! You're my little girl. What's the matter with you? (*She gets up and moves uncertainly toward Diana.*) I told my friends at the bar how nice you are.

At the touch of the woman, Diana bends her head—and her lips move as if a bad taste has suddenly come up her throat. Her face shows agony.

DIANA (*beginning to cry, in an imploring voice*): Please don't touch me . . .

"MOTHER": It's your father's fault. I'm sorry. He doesn't leave me money. He never does anything. The old bastard never does anything for us.

Diana stops crying. Compassion now shows through the tenseness on her face.

L.Y.: Change parts now. Reverse roles with your mother.

DIANA (*smiles, looking at the auxiliary ego playing her mother*): She's doing a great job.

Diana reverses roles and acts as her mother. She purses her lips, and her very slow delivery seems amazingly real.

DIANA AS MOTHER: Listen, don't you talk back to your mother like that. You're still my daughter and you're only six years old. You don't talk to me like that.

DIANA/MOTHER (*softens*): I know, baby. (She gets up and slowly goes to her as "Diana's" crying gets louder.) Ah yes! It's so miserable here. I know . . . this is a big terrible world. I know how you feel. I've tried to kill myself . . . so many times. I would just like to put my head in an oven and end it all. (Diana later reported that in reality, on several occasions the mother had attempted suicide by turning on the gas and putting her head in the oven.)

AUXILIARY EGO AS DIANA (*crying hysterically*): Don't tell me those things. I don't want to hear that.

I ask Diana in the role of the mother, "Why are you such an ineffectual mother?"

DIANA AS MOTHER: My mother was cruel to me. I never really had a father. He disappeared when I was a little kid.

Diana goes on in great detail in the role of her mother to explain why she is an alcoholic, and she begins to describe all of the confusion in her life, including the problems she is having with Diana's father.

(In hundreds of sessions I have directed, especially with adolescents who have had difficult childhoods, I note a strong [open or masked] hostility toward their parents. It is precisely this hostility that often defeats their own life. A technique I use is to place them in the role of their own parents. In this role I have them soliloquize why they, as their parent, are so cruel or ineffectual as parental socializing agents. Usually, they depict a parent who has had a most difficult and destructive childhood. Almost invariably, this process of confronting the difficult life their parent had, [in the role of the parent] relieves the enormous hostility that keeps the protagonist in trouble. I would recommend to everyone the simple technique of taking the role of your parent(s) and reviewing all of the negative and destructive experiences they have had. This process of comprehension will alleviate some of the negative feeling about your parent that often impairs your own life.)

L.Y.: All right, Diana, reverse roles and become yourself again.
DIANA (*as herself*): I understand what she's been through and I feel for her, but I'm crying because it still hurts me. At six I wasn't crying this much. It wouldn't have done me any good. (She was, no doubt, crying inside.)
L.Y.: Diana . . . now your father walks in (auxiliary ego father returns to center stage.)
DIANA (*looking at father*): I'm afraid of him. My mother and I leave a lot. Whenever she says, "I'm going to take my kid and get the hell out of here!" I'm really glad because I'm afraid of him.
L.Y.: You think he's going to kill her?
DIANA: I think he's going to kill me.
L.Y.: Does he hit you much?
DIANA: When he beats me up, I can hear my mother screaming in the background, "You're going to kill her, you're going to kill her."
L.Y.: What would he beat you up about?
DIANA: Oh . . . like . . . they were very weird. When they were together they worked in a defense plant, and my job was to clean the house when I came home from school. Once I stopped off at a friend's house and I didn't have the place all cleaned up by the time they got home. He took off his belt . . . and beat me with it.

He once really beat me badly when I was sixteen.

L.Y.: Okay, let's see that scene.

DIANA (*soliloquizing in Wayne's presence*) I'm sixteen. And I have a boyfriend. His name is Wayne. He's only seventeen but he's very mature for his age. He's really like a man. He is the only one who loves me . . . and I'm probably the only one who loves him. His parents don't give him anything. His father comes home from work and drinks beer and watches TV. His mother is kinda crazy. She just stares. It happened this one day Wayne came to take me out. I was putting on makeup and my father started yelling.

FATHER (*yelling*): Where you going?! You better stay in this house!

DIANA: I just want to step outside . . . for a minute . . .

FATHER: Goddamn it, I'll let you have it! . . .

DIANA: I run past him out of the door. And I go meet Wayne in a park near my house. I think I just sat on his lap. (*She does—and at once rests her head on his shoulder. Wayne embraces her.*) We always say, "What are we going to do? How are we going to get out of here?"

WAYNE: I've got to get you out of there. That place is killing you. We've got to go some place where we can be together. I miss you . . . I want to be with you all of the time. I love you so much. If that father of yours hits you again, I'll kill him. I'll get a fucking gun and I'll kill him!

DIANA: Please don't, please don't talk like that. We'll find another way. Maybe my mother will leave him pretty soon.

WAYNE: I'll have to get a car and some "bread," even if I have to steal. I've got to get you away from here.

DIANA: Don't, Wayne, please don't . . . I love you . . .

Diana finally goes home late that night. She reverses roles and plays her father. As the father, she punches "Diana" in the face. I have her play herself immediately after the punch.

DIANA (*as if she really felt the blow*): He broke my nose. (*Repeatedly, she touches her nose with both hands.*) I can see flashes . . . All I know is that my face . . . I get these flashes of light . . . And I know my eyes are starting to shut . . . and I can feel my face . . . I feel blood

L.Y.: What do you do?

DIANA: I fight him back. I kick him and I take an ashtray and hit him in the mouth with it.

For several minutes Diana thrashes around fighting with her "Father." She then goes to her room and sits alone holding her face.

L.Y.: What are you thinking? Just think out loud. Soliloquize.

DIANA (*holding both sides of her face with the flat of her hands*): I'm just glad to be alone. My nose is broken. (*Her chest heaves; she has difficulty catching her breath.*) I'm just lying here. I'm just glad that I'm away from them. And that I'm alive. (*She flexes her hands and moves her elbows.*) I think I'm all right. My face is pounding like . . . there is some blood . . . (*she touches her nose*) . . . but I'm all right. I'm glad it's over. I want to go to sleep. I'm really afraid. When they go to work tomorrow, Wayne is going to come to the house, and I know that if he sees my face, he's going to kill my father. He's going to get a gun and kill my father. I don't want Wayne to see me because he'll just get into trouble! The other day, he brought over a whole big bag of change. . . . I know he robbed some place. . . .

The next scene is set up with Wayne.

DIANA: I'm afraid every time you and your friends go out somewhere that you are going to get busted. You know . . . and I'm afraid that you're going to go to jail. And I don't want you to steal, I don't want you to take any cars. You're taking too much of a risk. I don't mind walking . . . I would rather walk ten miles. . . .

WAYNE: But I DO. There is nothing else I can do for you. I don't have any money.

DIANA: I'm telling you, Wayne . . . I don't mind. You always think that I have to have everything just so. You want to treat me like a queen . . . and you don't have anything. I don't mind. I just want to be with you. I don't care if I have to walk. Just so that we can be together. . . .

(*Diana has cued the auxiliary ego playing Wayne into his role.*)

WAYNE (*shaking his head*): It matters that when you're hungry I can't even buy you a hamburger. It matters when we have to walk ten fucking miles to my pad in the rain. I don't give a damn if I have to go and steal . . . It doesn't matter. I'm not going to get caught.

DIANA: You might.

WAYNE (*shaking his head*): No way. Don't worry, baby! You're my beautiful woman and we'll be together—forever.

DIANA: That's what I want. I don't even feel hunger when I am with you. Walking with you is the most fantastic thing in the world. I don't care if it is a hundred miles. I just like being with you. I don't feel any pain. I don't feel tired. I am just happy to be with you. YOU'RE THE ONLY PERSON I HAVE IN MY LIFE THAT I CARE ABOUT!!

Diana reveals the next event in her odyssey. She sits in the court-room and feels the pain of seeing Wayne sent to prison for stealing a car. She sobs at the loss as if he had died, because she never sees him again.

Right after he is sent away, she attempts to go to his house, to be near his clothes and possessions. Now all alone, she sits in her room in extreme pain, feeling totally alone. We set up the next scene.

DIANA: I'm in my bedroom. A bed, with a dresser and a mirror. I'm playing records. I'm playing Damita Joe. Damita Joe is singing a song called "Way Up High in the Sky." (*She begins to sing softly and in great pain.*) "There's a land in the sky and a place where we'll meet by and by. So dry your eyes, don't you cry. We will live all our dreams in the sky. When I look in your eyes, I see heaven and angels go by. So dream of our little love land. Land of ours way up high in the sky. I dreamed we were together. . . ." (*The pain is more than she can bear. She cries out.*) I can't stand to listen to it anymore. And it says, "We're alone in the sky." It's the only way we're going to be together—when we're dead! And I'm all alone all the time. I'm alone since Wayne went away. No one's here. No one cares about me. And I go in and look at the mirror and I . . . (*she lets out a scream and projects both hands forward*) . . . I break the mirror and destroy the room. (*She pounds on the wall with her hands to describe what she says.*) I take pieces of mirror and cut my arms . . . and I see the blood. Then I just want to die. Then I run out into the street. I don't care. I go up to this bar and I try to get drunk, but that doesn't do any good. It just makes me feel worse, and I go on like this for days and days. My parents are gone most of the time—out drunk. No one is ever at home. I wish I had the guts to kill myself, but I don't. So that's when I call up these guys.

L.Y.: What are their names?

DIANA (*closing her eyes to remember*): Wally was one . . . and a guy named Tommy.

Wally and Tommy take their positions on stage. They are both heroin addicts.

DIANA (*looking up at them*): I know you guys are using. Right? I want you to turn me on.

WALLY: What do you want to do that for?

DIANA: I just want to, that's all. I just want you to turn me on. That's all. I know what's happening. I know you guys are fixing. I know you're getting high. I've let you use my bathroom to fix.

You go in depressed and messed up and you come out looking like everything is cool.

WALLY: You'll get hooked.

DIANA: I don't know about getting hooked. I just know that I want to do what you're doing. I want to get high, and get out. I tried to get drunk and I really blew it. I got sick. That doesn't make it for me.

TOMMY: How do you know you want this?

DIANA (*determined*): I know I do. I know I do.

DIANA'S DOUBLE: It'll make me feel good.

DIANA: No! I just want to try it. I've made up my mind.

WALLY: All right, I'll . . .

DIANA (*interrupting him, remembering*): No, you tell me you're not going to.

WALLY: I really don't want to do it. You're too young. I'm cutting out.

DIANA (*fiercely*): You know what then? Don't ever come here anymore! Don't come to my house anymore. I don't want you at my pad. You're not going to use my bathroom anymore . . . to fix in. I don't ever want to see you again. Either turn me on or I want you to split.

WALLY: You're sure that's what you want?

DIANA (*grimly nodding her head*): I'm positive. That's what I want.

WALLY: Which arm do you want?

DIANA (*impatient*): I don't care.

L.Y.: Diana, as this is going on, I want you to think. What are you thinking?

Wally is holding her arm, looking for a vein. Tommy makes a tourniquet with his belt.

DIANA: I'm scared. But I feel so much emotional pain that I don't care. I wish I was dead anyway. So what's the difference? I don't care about anything.

Wally cooks up the dope. He strikes a match.

L.Y. (*I double for Diana*): Anything has got to be better than the way I feel. I've tried suicide . . . (*pause*) . . . right? . . . I got to get out.

DIANA: I don't care what happens to me. I'm scared, but I don't care what happens. I have nothing to live for. I want more than anything to get out, to get away from my feelings.

Wally simulates fixing her with an injection of heroin. Diana ACTUALLY looks as if she has just received a jolt of heroin.

She, of course, knows the feeling. She appears very relaxed. Members of the group smile, because they know the feeling. (Diana at this point was so mesmerized by the session and so into her feelings that she later told me the psychodramatic fix almost felt like a real fix of heroin.)

DIANA: Oh, wow. (*She bends her head back; her face seems very peaceful but her mouth twists.*) I feel kind of nauseated. I feel good. I feel very, very relaxed. (*She sort of half smiles.*) Hey, you know what? (*She opens her eyes.*) I really don't care about anything anymore. (She repeats it with more assurance and quietly closes her eyes.) I really don't care. (*She leans her head back.*) I really feel cool.

WALLY AND TOMMY: You know, baby, you're with us now. Like you're a hope-to-die junkie . . . and, you know, life's going to be good. All you got to do is score . . . and you feel good.

DIANA: Yeah. I feel good. I feel good. I don't have any more fear or pain. I'm out of my misery. Even my love for Wayne seems like a dream. Something unreal or that happened a long time ago.

It is apparent that Diana's journey into dope was a way of relieving her emotional pain. The other members of the group of ex-addicts completely understand her trip and relate their own experiences and motivations. Diana and the group agree that they are now exploring their pain rather than trying to escape from it, because they agree that the "escape" into drugs (or alcohol) is, in the final analysis, more deadly and destructive than their original problems.

Rehearsal for Life

Psychodramas can be useful in preparation for life roles that are *necessary* for an individual's effective participation in society. One specific area where it has been found useful is in preparing parolees and recently released mental patients for participation in necessary roles and life situations. The parolee from an institution must find and maintain a job as a necessary condition of his release, whether he likes it or not. The mental patient on release, if he is to function, must be equipped in some minimal way to operate in everyday situations.

In another context, when a couple divorces, or a husband dies, the wife may have to adjust to a new life. For example she may have to go job hunting, perhaps for the first time in her life. Psychodrama can help prepare her for new adjustments. In brief, I will present here some extreme cases of adjustment that exemplify the problems most people confront on a less extreme level. In this sense, most people in their lives at some point are "parolees" or "ex-patients" attempting to enter a new way of life. You can attempt to identify with these cases in that context.

Although a person starting a new life may have a fear and anxiety that is rooted in more complex psychological dynamics, it is still absolutely necessary that a person must be prepared to act effectively in key areas of their new social life. Psychodrama and role-playing can often cut through the complexity of an individual's personality problem and help prepare him for required situations, as a kind of rehearsal for life.

In this analysis, we will focus on parolees leaving prison and entering a new life, although, as indicated, the approach would be applicable to others starting out anew.

Although it is recognized that a person may require more intense therapeutic attention, "getting by" vital situations is an important wedge to keep him interacting on the "normal" social scene, where a favorable life position may produce therapeutic results. In brief, the individual, once he or she is "in action," can flourish, in contrast with someone who has no starting point. Rehearsing "core" situations in psychodrama can get the person going.

The procedure for helping a parolee or a person entering a new life style involves several steps: (1) With the cooperation of the subject, we select key "future" situations and roles that he has to play and that he feels inadequate to perform; (2) we project the subject into the situations with the aid of auxiliary egos, role reversal, doubles, and other psychodramatic techniques that seem indicated; (3) we follow up with the subject of the session on his performance in actual situations; and (4) we use psychodramatic procedures to have the subject further explore these situations and reinforce his positive actions.

The following case illustrates the application of psychodrama to one person in this context. Jack was a fifty-year-old parolee recently released from a state prison. In his lifetime, he had spent more time in correctional institutions than in the open community. His offenses included narcotics addiction, assault, and robbery.

He came to my attention as a member of a group with whom I was meeting weekly in an effort to help them become better integrated into their jobs and the community. With Jack and the group, it was determined that two basic key roles and situations necessary for Jack to maintain were (1) his job and (2) reporting to his parole officer.

Jack role-played a number of situations on his job with members of the group playing auxiliary roles. The major problem for Jack in this area was the big gap between his conception of what was adequate performance on the job and that of his employer. Slowly, Jack began to accept the fact that perhaps many of the gripes he had were not valid. Although he still felt he was right, he agreed that he would have to accept his employer's view of his performance, since the job was a necessary condition for his remaining in the community.

The second key role that he abhorred was the necessity of reporting to his parole officer. After a number of sessions in which he acted this out, Jack accepted more fully the fact that he had to report or he would be returned to prison.

Role reversal was most effective in this situation. Jack, while playing the role of his parole officer, soliloquized, "This guy needs to report somewhere at least once a week so that he can be reminded that he is on parole and that if he fouls up one more time we're going to lock him up and throw away the key. Maybe I don't really do him any good with his problems, because I'm so busy with a big case load, but he has to come in regularly or else." The group at first sided with Jack and his attitude of "why report, it doesn't do me any good"; however, after considerable psycho-dramatic exploration, they reinforced Jack's conclusion that it was essential and probably useful for him to report to his parole officer.

Although the sessions did not greatly reorganize Jack's basic personality structure, they did help him to accept two essential conditions necessary for his remaining outside the walls. This enabled him to remain in relationship with a group whose understanding of him and his problems put them in a position to be therapeutic agents. The sessions were instrumental in placing Jack in a favorable sociometric position where it was possible for him in day-to-day *in situ* interaction to receive successful therapeutic action.

As indicated, a psychodramatic rehearsal for life has other applications. People freshly divorced are confronted with a variety of new, challenging, and sometimes fearful situations, including dating, relating to their children under different circumstances, new financial issues, a different sexual pattern or orientation, and the realignment of their former relationship with their spouse. People in a new job find psychodrama a useful rehearsal for their work situation. In brief, without necessarily going into intensive psychodynamic depth, a psychodrama can provide a rehearsal for a new life situation.

A Psychodramatic Suicide

Many people at critical points in their life have considered suicide. Most people do not commit the act, but many harbor the thought and there are insidious personal consequences. Their psyche festers with the consideration of this alternative. We have found through many sessions on this subject that people are relieved of their conflict about "to be or not to be" after a good session.

Directing a psychodramatic suicide is a delicate matter. Enacting suicide in psychodrama may have the therapeutic impact of saving a life; however, it is obviously a scenario that must be approached with the greatest caution, since it could backfire.

As I was warming up to a psychodrama session at a state hospital with a group of patients, I noticed a man of about thirty, about six feet tall, slender, fragile-looking, who had fresh bandages on his wrists. I asked him if he wanted a session. He assented and came forward.

L.Y.: Would you introduce yourself to the group?

BARNEY: My name is Barney, I'm thirty-one, and this is an unusual situation for me. For three years I have been a male nurse at ———— State Hospital. Last week I attempted suicide, and I'm now here as a patient.

L.Y.: Before we proceed, Barney—that is, if we do proceed—let me present to you the psychodramatic rationale for a session on suicide. We can assume several things: the "to be or not to be" question is something that consciously or unconsciously is in the mind of many people who never make the attempt. There is some hazard in having this session because it will revive memories and feelings related to your attempt on your life. Our guiding theme in psychodrama is, however, that when you attempted your act of suicide you had no support from anyone. You felt completely alienated and alone . . .

BARNEY: That's true.

L.Y.: You obviously can't fully relive the scenario here, but we can stage it in terms of your memory. Only this time you will have others—this group—*support you* through your crisis. Also, we may be able to provide some insights into the forces that drove you to the act. On this basis, do you feel like proceeding? It's clearly your choice.

BARNEY: Okay. Let's go.

L.Y.: Obviously, the background to your suicide attempt goes back many years. However, for now, let's focus on the time period immediately preceding your attempt.

BARNEY: Well, about ten hours or so before I cut my wrists I was drinking with a couple of people (*he adds with hostility and sarcasm*) who I thought were my friends.

L.Y.: Okay, let's go back to that point in time. Set up the scene—time, place, and all that.

BARNEY: Well, it *was* about 5:00 p.m.

L.Y.: No. *It is* 5:00 p.m.

BARNEY: Okay. It's 5:00 p.m. and I'm home in my apartment. It's a two-bedroom—not bad. (*He looks around, sets up chairs on stage.*)

L.Y.: Who else is there at the time?

BARNEY (*with anger*): My supposed girlfriend, Sandy, and my best friend, Bob. See, she's been living with me for about six months. We even thought of getting married.

L.Y.: Does Bob live there?

BARNEY: Well, he kind of crashes here, once in a while. And when things aren't going good, he stays awhile. He's been here now for a week.

L.Y.: Okay. Here's Bob and Sandy. (*Two people from the group are selected as auxiliary egos.*) You're all drinking pretty good? (*Yeah.*) Okay, go over on the side and fill them in briefly on the situation. (*After a few minutes*): Don't go into too many details, just get into the essence of the scene. Go ahead, Barney.

BARNEY: I'm going to come right out and say it. I think you two have been fucking around when I'm not here!

BOB: Christ, Barney, how can you say that to a pal?

BARNEY: Some pal. You son-of-a-bitch. I know.

SANDY: Oh, there you go again with your jealous bullshit. I don't like being accused like this.

BARNEY: I just know it's true!

> *This goes on for several minutes with denials and accusations. Finally, there's a brief truce called, and they all decide to go out to dinner. The drinking continues. The scene in the restaurant, according to Barney, gets very sloppy. Finally, they're back at the apartment, still arguing.*

BARNEY (*cajoling*): Come on, Sandy, just admit it. I don't care. It's okay with me. Christ, I'm no prude. Anything goes—these days.

SANDY (*finally*): Okay, if you really want to know, we have made it a few times. So what!

> *Barney is crushed. I stop the action and give him a double. Between them they reveal how distraught they are.*

BARNEY (*crying*): I feel like the only two people in the world who meant anything to me have deserted me. My mom and dad are both dead. These two were the only family I had. I feel completely smashed.

L.Y.: What happens next?

BARNEY: Well, we make peace. I acted like I accepted it—which, of course, I didn't. I continued drinking and got so drunk I passed out on my bed.

L.Y.: Okay. What happens next?

Barney lies on floor (bed) with his double. It's the middle of the night, around 3:00 a.m.

BARNEY (*stretching*): I've been drinking a lot, so I get up to go to the bathroom.

DOUBLE: I wonder where Sandy and Bob are.

BARNEY: I have an idea, but don't want to know.

DOUBLE: Well, we better go look.

BARNEY: I really don't want to, but I can't stop myself.

They walk to the other bedroom.

L.Y.: What do you see?

Barney stands in the bedroom doorway.

BARNEY: There they are, the two bastards—in bed nude. They've probably just made it and they're asleep. Bob must hear me. He opens his eyes—for a second—then acts like he's sleeping.

We have Bob and Sandy lying in front of him curled up together and sleeping.

L.Y.:Soliloquize your feelings as you look at them.

BARNEY: I feel pain in my gut. I feel a heaviness. I'm betrayed. I'm all alone in the world. No one cares. I'll show those bastards. I'll show everyone. The thought flashes in my mind of "getting them." Then I decide—I'll just get out myself. I can't stand the pain.

He goes to the bathroom, gets a razor blade, and cuts his wrists.

L.Y.: What are you thinking?

BARNEY: Now someone will have to pay attention to me. They'll feel sorry for what *they* made me do.

L.Y.: Say it again.

BARNEY (*screaming*): NOW SOMEONE WILL HAVE TO PAY ATTENTION TO ME!!

To reinforce what Barney says, I have everyone in the group chant in loud voices three times: "NOW SOMEONE WILL HAVE TO PAY ATTENTION TO ME!!"

It is obvious at this point that everyone in the group is "paying attention" and is deeply affected by Barney's session. In the post-discussion, around half of the group talks about their feelings at different times in their lives about suicide. Several had actually made the attempt. There is an outpouring of emotions about being alone and uncared for. Several people come up and hug Barney.

L.Y. How do you feel right now, Barney?

BARNEY: I feel good. I've been worrying about this since I've been in the hospital. My fear has been: Will I try it again? Now, I don't think I will. In fact, this has been like trying it again—only all of you were with me and it wasn't so bad.

I guess I picked a couple of losers as friends—but I know everyone isn't like those two creeps.

I have a good feeling since I learned a lot of other people once
felt like I did. Of course, I learned this in my work, but I really
believe it today. Maybe this "attempt" takes care of it for me. I
know I really want to live.

Certainly, there are other dynamics to Barney's personality that
brought him to suicide, and he, of course, required more extensive
psychotherapy. The session, however, gave him an opportunity to
explore his suicide, with the assistance of the group. It was not
necessary to overtly articulate every insight he received. Much of
what Barney learned took place within the action of his powerful
session. Acting-out suicide (or homicide) in a psychodramatic
context provides the opportunity to perform the act without the
horrendous and final consequences of the real life act. The protagonist can learn about his motivations in action and, therefore,
may be deterred from acting-out destructively in life.

Again, this is a delicate psychodramatic session and should
only be performed in the presence of a compassionate group by a
skilled director with considerable experience.

On Death and Dying

In psychodrama one readily becomes aware that people can
fixate on many aspects of life, and in many cases on death. In
some instances, a dead person can become more important in the
consciousness of an individual than those people who are alive
and with whom he interacts daily.

This tends to occur most often when a person dies toward
whom the protagonist has some extreme emotional feeling that
has not been expressed during their life. The feeling may be
strong love or hatred (sometimes both), and the protagonist during his lifetime never felt able to tell the other person how he felt.

In some cases, the spouse who is the survivor of a death feels hostility. As one female protagonist, Carol, stated, "I know it's irrational, but I'm furious with you for dying and deserting me." In this case, the survivor wife had another unresolved and un-expressed emotion: "When you were alive I was a dependent housewife, without any identity of my own. Since you died I have really become somebody. I have a good job, take care of the kids, and I've become a real person. I really love you and it hurts me that you've never seen me this way. Another thing I wish I could tell you about is how guilty I feel every time I go out with an-other man. I feel like I'm betraying our love. The thing that hurts me most is that because of these mixed feelings, I feel too guilty to enjoy the beautiful memories of the happy times we spent to-gether." The psychodrama experience of Carol, with the aid of a perceptive double, telling her husband (played by an auxiliary ego) about all of these emotions was painful—but liberating. As Carol insightfully stated after her session: "I still love him, but I've never really confronted these feelings. Maybe now I can let him go, enjoy my memories, and go on with life." Several other people present at the session expressed parallel situations and emotions. This seemed to help Carol feel she was not alone and facilitated freeing her from her complex negative emotions.

In brief, many emotions felt by survivors toward the dead per-son often remain unresolved and require psychodramatic expres-sion and clarification. Another example of this problem relates to a suicide in which the deceased left a vicious note for his survivor, loading her with guilt about his death. The dead husband in a peculiar way had the "last word"—and the survivor was left with a painful package of unresolved feelings of guilt and grief. Her psychodrama was useful, especially when her psycho-dramatic husband and the group absolved her of any guilt for the husband's act.

In another context, "social death," as, for example, in "the death of a marriage," one or both parties may be left frustrated with unresolved feeling because the partner leaves suddenly and does not provide any opportunity for dialogue.

We find, in psychodrama, that even one production with an auxiliary ego playing the role of the deceased relieves the sense of guilt or frustration felt by the protagonist. It is often amazing to note the great and persistent emotions felt toward the dead by most people.

In a prototypical session on this subject, a woman, Mary, came forward and told how her life had been hell since her husband had died in an automobile crash. They had been married ten years. She opened the session of her husband's death by telling how they had quarreled just before he left the house for his fatal automobile trip.

She psychodramatically entered into the scene, the evening of his death. They argued about something. She couldn't even remember the subject of their conflict. He ran out the door in anger. She did not try to stop him.

MARY: (*now alone with her double*): Well, he's gone—but he'll be back.
MARY'S DOUBLE: Why do I start trouble. I really love Joe.
MARY: Yes, I love him. But I haven't been able to tell him so for years. We just seem to be at each other all the time.
MARY'S DOUBLE: It's mostly my fault that we fight. I'm afraid of love and dependency.
MARY: That's true. It seems like I have to keep things boiling and our relationship on the edge of disaster. I hate myself for doing this, because Joe is the sweetest person in the world. He's my only and best friend.
   Phone rings. Mary picks it up.
MARY (*to me*): I can't do this.
L.Y.: I think you should go through it, Mary. Maybe we can exorcize your pain.
MARY (*continuing*): Hello, who's this?
VOICE: Mary Rhodes?
MARY: Yes.
VOICE: This is the police. I regret to inform you your husband was just killed in a car crash.
   Masy breaks into deep sobs. Her double puts her arms around her. She sobs for several minutes, then seems to calm down.
L.Y.: Soliloquize your feelings, Mary.

MARY: Oh, my God. Why did this happen to me? I *know* that if I had been kinder and let Joe know how much I loved him, this would never have happened. It's my fault! It's my fault!

I set up the next scene, in which she talks to her dead husband. Mary claims, half in humor through her tears, that the scene must take place in heaven.

MARY: Joe, I know we would still be together if I wasn't such a bitch.

JOE: How can you blame yourself like this? It could have happened to anyone—any time.

MARY: No. I KNOW IN MY HEART THAT IT WASN'T AN ACCIDENT. IT WAS SUICIDE. YOU WANTED TO DIE BECAUSE OF MY CRUELTY.

Mary begins to sob again. She reveals that she had never consciously thought that it was suicide until she expressed it in the psychodrama. She continues with Joe.

JOE: Mary, why are you torturing yourself with guilt? It wasn't suicide—it WAS an accident.

MARY: If I could only believe that.

I have the group join in, chanting several times: "It was an accident, not suicide."

MARY: Whatever happened, Joe. I want you to know that I love you and have beautiful memories of our being together.

They embrace, and Joe tells Mary he always loved her, too.

JOE: Now you have to let go. Put me in the past where I belong. You're still young and beautiful. You can find a new life.

MARY: It's hard to let go. I've thought of nothing but you since you died. But I'll try.

JOE: Forgive yourself. You did nothing wrong.

In subsequent sessions, Mary "forgave" herself and we later learned that Mary did give up the past. She began to date and eventually remarried.

In the post-discussion of Mary's session, several people "made peace" with the dead people *in their lives.* One young man kissed his "mother" and told her how much he loved her. A young woman raged in her encounter with her dead father about how much she hated him. After she told him and expressed her hostility, she forgave him for not being a good father. The resolution of these often unexpressed feelings invariably produces a sense of peacefulness in the people who work out these complex emotions about death through psychodrama.

The Psychodrama of Birth

For many people, having a child is one of the most beautiful, significant, and awesome acts of their life. Despite the positive emotions, there are often a myriad of normal doubts that also arise in the process. Do I want my spouse as the father or mother? Am *I* capable of being a good father or mother? Do I want a boy or a girl, and why? Do I want the child at all? Many psychodrama sessions revolve around these issues of "having a child."

In one prototype session, a young lady came on stage. She is two months pregnant. After some preliminary introductory scenes, she gets to the center of her problem.

JUNE: Ralph and I were on the verge of splitting up when I found myself pregnant. The doctor told me my diaphragm wasn't foolproof, and he was right. This is a child that we're not sure we want, and we have to come to a decision in a few weeks, or I understand having an abortion becomes more difficult to perform.
L.Y.: I know Ralph is here, but I'm going to have someone stand in for him as an auxiliary ego. Where do you discuss this matter?
JUNE: Where else? In bed.
L.Y.: Okay. Set it up. You and Ralph are in bed. Get into the mood of the situation. Describe the furniture, the colors in the room. Which side of the bed do you sleep on?
   June sets up the situation with the auxiliary ego playing Ralph. She describes her surroundings in detail. This is helpful in warming up both June and the group to the situation.
JUNE: Well, what should we do?
"RALPH": I think you should have the abortion. It's really very easy these days . . .
JUNE (*breaks into tears*): You don't love me—or you'd want our baby.
"RALPH": Loving you has nothing to do with it. Christ, I can hardly afford to feed us. We just aren't ready now.
JUNE (*crying and bitter*): Okay. It's your decision. I think we could make it okay. But if that's what you want.
RALPH (*furiously*): That's what drives me up a wall. Everything is my decision or my fault. Screw it—I don't want total responsibility anymore. You take some responsibility for yourself.

L.Y.: Is that the way he acts?

JUNE: Exactly!

We note in the group that the real Ralph has a weak smile on his face and begins to squirm in his seat.

L.Y.: Okay, June. I'm sure you've never done this before, but in psychodrama your fetus can talk.

We set up the situation with an auxiliary ego, representing the third person in the life situation, kneeling in front of June on the stage.

L.Y.: Is it a girl or a boy?

JUNE: If it was a boy, that would be fine. But I'm afraid it's a girl.

FETUS: Hello, Mommy. Do you love me?

JUNE: Of course I love you. But you scare me.

FETUS: Why do I scare you?

JUNE: I'm afraid you're going to turn out like me and you'll suffer a lot like I did.

FETUS: I'm really nice, Mommy. I'll be a cute little girl and I'll be very sweet. Please don't kill me.

JUNE (*sobbing*): I don't want to. But I'm afraid your Daddy will leave and then we'll be alone. I can't take care of you alone. I'm afraid.

FETUS: Don't be afraid. We'll have fun. It'll be great.

JUNE (*angry*): No! I'm just getting my own identity as a woman. I'll be finishing college soon and I don't want a burden.

FETUS (*puts its arms around her*): Please, Mommy.

The real Ralph begins to cry and comes on stage. He puts his arms around June and the "girl."

RALPH: Please don't cry, June. We'll make it. You know I really love you. I want the child.

JUNE: But it's so hard to live in this world. Should we really bring another human being into this mess?

L.Y.: Okay, June, move over. Ralph, you talk to your unborn child.

Ralph kneels down and kisses June's stomach.

RALPH: First of all, you're a boy and your name is Mike. And listen, Mike, you're going to be the greatest guy that ever lived. We'll play ball together and go out to the country. We'll really have fun.

I have to tell you, though, there's a lot of crap in the world. There's poverty and crooked politicians and corruption. The air is full of smog. But even so, you're going to be a great man and help change things. And I'll help you.

June and Ralph embrace. Apparently, they have made their decision. At this point, various members of the group are very involved. Others come up to express their feelings about having a child. Some reflect great fear and negativity about bringing up a child in the contemporary world.

One lady chooses this opportunity to talk to her nine-year-old daughter:

MARGIE: Your dad is gone and sometimes you are an awful pain in the ass. But you mean everything to me. Honestly. I've often regretted having you. But I don't know what I would do without you. I love you very much. And I want to tell June here: Have your child. There's no other experience like it.

The group, continuing into the post-discussion, reflects varied feelings and opinions about this significant and intense experience.

The psychodrama of birth is a session I would suggest to every couple contemplating the birth of a child. A psychodrama director can be helpful but is not necessary. The expectant couple plus at least one friend are required for the session. In turn, the potential father and mother assume their anticipated parental role. Another member of the group plays the role of a son or daughter, depending on the choice of the protagonist. Some suggested questions from the auxiliary ego "child" are: "Do you really want me? What kind of world am I being born into? Do you love me? I know you want a boy (or girl)—what if I'm the wrong sex, how will you feel about me? When I grow up, what kind of work would you ideally like me to do? Will you spend a lot of time with me?" Next we would have the parent take the role of the child and see himself from that perspective.

Childhood Injustices—Religious Hypocrisy

Many people live out their lives deeply affected by a childhood experience. Sometimes a child is subject to a series of injustices. In many cases, this sense of injustice negatively dominates their life. This has been revealed in several of the sessions already presented. The following psychodrama delineates another aspect of this issue.

L.Y. (in the warm-up): In our group tonight, people have varying levels of religious belief. Some of you have expressed interest in doing a psychodrama of God. Those of you who believe in God have varying ideas or concepts of what *your* God is like. Is your concept male or female? Is your God love, or is It an avenging fire and brimstone God?

PERSON 1: I wish you existed, God, but you don't. If you exist, why do you let good people die in accidents? Why do children starve? Why do you let good people die from disease? If you exist, you're cruel and arbitrary.

PERSON 2: Oh, Lord, you are pure love to me. I never question the imponderables. I just believe in you and I'm saved. How can people question your existence? You're in every beautiful living thing. Praise the Lord.

In the group, a woman of around forty, named Rachel, begins to sob.

L.Y.: What is it, Rachel?

RACHEL: I have faith, but it's tarnished. I go to church regularly and I want to believe—but it's hard.

L.Y.: Come up here and talk to your God.

She steps up on the stage.

RACHEL: Oh, Lord, I think you're wonderful, but how could you let such a terrible thing happen to a little innocent girl!

L.Y.: What happened, Rachel?

RACHEL: Well, it happened when I was only around eleven years old—just an innocent little girl.

L.Y.: Where were you? Set up the scene.

RACHEL: Here I am, playing on the porch at my grandparents'. I'm here for the weekend because my parents had to go somewhere.

L.Y.: Okay, here you are on the porch. Just soliloquize.

RACHEL (*in a little girl's voice*): Well, I'm all alone because my grandmother went shopping. I'm here with my grandpa, who is also the preacher in our church. I don't like him too much. He always looks at me funny. He never smiles.

I send in "Grandpa." He walks over and just glowers at the girl.

RACHEL: Let me play him.

She reverses roles and becomes the grandpa.

RACHEL AS GRANDPA: What are you doing? Look at you, you

wicked, sinful girl. You're sitting there with your legs open. I can see your panties!

RACHEL: I'm sorry, Grandpa.

RACHEL AS GRANDPA: You're sorry! The devil must have hold of a nasty little girl like you. I'll fix you.

Rachel as grandpa simulates taking her pants down and spanking her on her bare bottom. We reverse roles.

RACHEL (*crying*): Please, grandpa, don't. I'll be good! I'll be good.

GRANDPA (*continues*): I'll fix you.

He simulates what Rachel claims actually happened. He takes a stick and inserts it in her vagina, then he uses his fingers to masturbate her. Rachel is in tears, ashamed and frightened.

RACHEL: Please, grandpa. No! No! It hurts!

GRANDPA: I'll get the devil out of there. (*Finally, relieved in some way*): Rachel, this is between you, me, and God. If you ever tell anyone about this you will be punished terribly. The devil will take you straight to hell!

RACHEL: I won't tell anyone, Grandpa.

L.Y.: How do you feel this moment? You're still eleven.

RACHEL: I'm scared to death and I'm humiliated. I hate him because I don't believe anything he said. I know he did something awful to me and I better not tell anyone.

L.Y.: Do you?

RACHEL: Yes, about a week later I try to tell my mother.

We set up the scene with "Mother."

RACHEL: Mom, I want to tell you something.

MOM: Yes, Rachel. What is it?

RACHEL: Well, when you and Dad were gone, Grandpa did something to me.

MOM (*suspicious*): What on earth are you talking about?

RACHEL: Well, he put a stick, then his fingers, in here.

We have Rachel reverse roles and become her mother, so we will have the actual *response of the mother.*

RACHEL AS MOM (*begins to shake her*): You disgusting little girl. You're just making that up. Tell me you're just making that up, or you'll get the worst beating of your life.

RACHEL (*crying*): But he did, Momma!

We have Rachel return to her own role.

  "Mother" starts to beat Rachel by punching a pillow held in front of Rachel.

MOM: Take that and that. Now you tell me you're lying!

RACHEL (*finally, in tears*): Okay, okay, Mom. I made it up.

MOM (*stops hitting her*): How could you possibly say that about your own grandpa. He's a minister of God and a deacon in the church. You nasty girl. Go to your room. You have a dirty mind.

In her room, Rachel and her double soliloquize the extreme pain of their feeling of injustice and being alone in the world with a terrible, "shameful" unsharable secret.

L.Y.: What happens next?

RACHEL: Not much, except on Sundays I have to go to church and I have to sit there week after week hearing my hypocrite Grandfather preach about God, love, and fire and brimstone. I felt like vomiting. I've lived with this feeling for forty years.

We set up a scene in which she talks to God again. We have a woman in the group who is in reality an ordained minister play God.

RACHEL: Well, that's it. How can I believe in you after that?

GOD: Just because one of my servants is sick and is a hypocrite, this shouldn't destroy your faith in me.

This goes back and forth with the real minister from the group playing God. In the final scene, we role-play having God remove the grandfather from the ministry. Rachel vents her extreme aggression by "beating" the minister grandfather with a battoca. We then psychodramatically have the grandfather get up in front of the entire congregation, recant, and personally apologize to Rachel.

GOD: Rachel is a wonderful girl—she never did anything wrong. It was all her grandfather's fault. (To mother): You should have believed your daughter.

Everyone in the group, including the "mother" and "grandfather," comes forward and extolls Rachel's virtues and apologizes for having hurt her all these years. Rachel beams throughout this scene, wherein she is fully vindicated by "psychodramatic justice."

L.Y.: Can you forgive him?

RACHEL: I'll try. (Pauses) No, I really can't—at least, not right now. And I can't forgive my mother either for all the pain I've felt. I can understand how God's servants can be corrupt. I accept that it's not God's fault, and that makes me feel a little better.

It has been an emotional session, not only for Rachel but also for the group. After the formal post-discussion of sharing, the group remained for several hours informally discussing the session and its personal meaning to various members of the group.

Rachel told me a few weeks after the session that it was very valuable to her. She had talked to a few people about the experience over the years, but this was the first time she had openly revealed it before a group. She felt the group's supportive and affectionate response was very therapeutic.

Over the years, I have run many sessions related to childhood injustices. In another session, a man of forty-five, now a psychiatrist, recalled a situation that occurred when he was seven. He had been beaten unjustifiably by a sadistic priest-schoolteacher in his homeland of Austria when he was a child. The psychiatrist had never resolved his extreme feelings of pain, humiliation, and injustice, although he had considerable therapy, including long-term psychoanalysis. In psychodrama he located his pain, felt it, retaliated against the schoolteacher, and, finally, partially forgave the man who had inflicted the injustice on him. The incident had left severe emotional scars, which were partially ameliorated by the psychodrama group process.

Correcting Life

In terms of our personal standards, we are often imperfect actors in life and we live to regret our mistakes. The just-missed love affair, the failed effort to properly tell off an "enemy," and the bungled opportunity to tell someone you love them are all examples of unfulfilled actions that produce a sense of frustration that often continues to plague peoples' life.

Psychodrama provides the opportunity and the vehicle for exacting these frustrations. We have had sessions with people who turned down a job and then acted-out how it might have been if they had taken it. In another session, a man stayed with his wife when he wanted to run off with another woman. He ran off with the other woman psychodramatically, and after an extensive session concluded that he really made the right decision and that it would have been a disaster if he had left with the other woman. Many people live out their lives with painful unresolved situations, as indicated by a variety of sessions. A frequent situation is the frustration of being oppressed and rejected as a child and never having the opportunity to hit back.

In one session, a man came on stage and began to enact a number of childhood scenes with a hated stepfather. In a crucial scene of his scenario, at the age of seven he was spanked by his stepfather with his mother present.

He gets into the scene. As he's in the simulated position of being beaten by an auxiliary ego stepfather, he soliloquizes:

TOM (*crying*): You dirty son-of-a-bitch. You vicious bastard, beating a little kid. I didn't even do anything that bad. I'll get you some day. I'll make you pay for this pain and humiliation. Mom, please stop him.

"MOTHER": I can't do anything. I'm stuck with him. I don't like what he does but I have to put up with him. We both need him to take care of us, no matter now he does it.

TOM: I know, Mom. I understand why you have to put up with him. But I'll get him someday.

L.Y.: Do you get even with him?

TOM: In a way.

L.Y.: Show us.

TOM: Well, we finally left the bastard. My mother remarried, a pretty nice guy. But I never forgot or forgave my stepfather, Harold. As you know, I'm a salesman and I travel a lot. Well, one day around five years ago, I was back East and I was in the town where we used to live. I tracked down my stepfather's address through a relative. And I was happily on my way to beat the shit out of the son-of-a-bitch. Remember, I carried this hatred and frustration with me for over twenty years.

L.Y.: Okay, set it up. You're in front of the building where he lives. Soliloquize your feelings.

TOM: Well, here I am. I'm finally going to get him. I'll just beat him up badly. I don't want to kill him even if he deserves it, because I don't want to screw myself up.

   (*Tom in the session is perspiring and actually nervously shaking with rage.*)

I walk into this dilapidated apartment building. And there's the buzzer. Harold J——. I'm in a cold sweat. I feel both fear and anger. The buzzer opens the door. I walk up two flights and I'm in front of his door.

L.Y.: Okay, hold it there a minute. Soliloquize.

We have Tom soliloquize his thoughts in this crucial moment so he can gather together his feelings, and also for the purpose of getting him more fully in the mood for his impending encounter.

TOM (*in summary, his soliloquy reveals*): I'm here and I'm going to get him. I'm scared but I feel good about acting-out my feelings.

L.Y.: Okay. The door opens and there he is.

HAROLD: Hello? Can I help you?

TOM: I'm thinking I can't believe my eyes. It's him all right. I recognize the face. But he's a little, old, skinny man living in this dump of an apartment. I can't beat him up. In one way he's the guy, but in another way he's a different person from the one I have hated all these years.

HAROLD: Yes?

TOM: Oh. Don't you remember me? It's Tom.

HAROLD: Tom? Oh, for Christ's sake. Tom Taylor. Jeezus, you're a big guy now. Come on in, son. Would you like a beer?

TOM: I go in and sit down and I still feel angry. Imagine him calling me "son" after all the beatings he gave me. But then he says something that wipes me out.

L.Y.: Reverse roles. Be him.

TOM AS HAROLD: Well, my boy. You look like you're getting along fine. How's your mother?

"TOM": Okay. How are you doing?

TOM AS HAROLD: Well, not so hot. I've had a few heart attacks, and the doctors tell me I don't have too long to go.

After some further small talk, Tom winds it up. "Well, I didn't get him—but how could I?"

Others in the group ventilate similar frustrations, when they were unable to consummate lingering frustrations and hostilities. Others successfully act out in the present situations that were sources of frustration or non-fulfillment for many years.

Psychodrama provides the opportunity for correcting or filling in some of the gaps of real life. People injured, rejected, or oppressed in the past can psychodramatically resolve these feelings in a session in the present. In effect, they are dealing with the monodrama on their thought level that has plagued them for years.

Psychodrama provides an opportunity to objectify the scene in action with the required cast of characters in the "here and now."

In one sense, as in all psychodrama, the protagonist is *not* going into the past. He or she is living in the present with a certain set of emotions that have their own reality. No one can ever totally recapitulate the actual scene from the past. But one can very effectively and usefully investigate his "here and now" perception of a frustrating scenario from the past. In most cases, the protagonist's enactment of the frustration and correction of his past life in psychodrama is beneficial to him.

Psychodrama Exercises

Some psychodrama exercises are suggested by the "correcting life" issue for possible enactments with a group of friends. (The more expanded use of psychodrama in this way in impromptu groups is more fully explicated in Chapter V.) The group, ideally, should be comprised of approximately six to eight people who know each other quite well. The members of the group should, of course, trust each other, and have some background in leveling honestly with each other. At first the group warm-up should take the form of each group member, in sequence, soliloquizing for three to five minutes a core situation of frustration, perhaps in their marriage, or a childhood injustice. Then each member should have the opportunity to select the person they want to direct their session and the person or persons who play the key role in their core situation. The protagonist should then have ten to fifteen minutes to act out the problem situation as it happened to him. After completing the problem situation, the protagonist should have the opportunity to act out the same situation as he wishes it had happened. For example, in the sessions presented here, young Rachel would first act out the traumatic situation with the preacher, then her corrective session might be one when the minister admits his crime against her, and finally her mother would completely believe in her and sympathize with the assault that was inflicted on her. In Tom's session, after he presented the scenes in which he was beaten as a child, he would have a "corrective scene" in which his mother apologized for permitting the stepfather to beat him. Also, the stepfather would admit he had problems and that Tom was a good boy, and he would apologize for the assaults.

There are a myriad of other possibilities for using psychodrama in impromptu groups. For example, a psychodramatic exercise could be utilized in the impromptu group to ascertain potential parent's emotions about pregnancy and the birth of a child. In another case, somewhat less emotional and traumatic, a man would enact a scene in which he was humiliated by an employer. In the corrective scene, he would cathart his frustration to forcefully answering back.

In brief, (1) the core problem or frustration scene is acted out, then (2) the protagonist corrects the negative scene by acting-out in a positive one that *he* delineates. This gives him the opportunity to correct a trauma. In hundreds of sessions I have directed where this is done, most all protagonists have experienced a sense of catharsis, and the corrective session has relieved the burden of carrying the problem around in their psyche. A clearer understanding of the variety of psychodramatic methods and techniques and their rationale in specific situations is a requisite for the proper application of psychodrama.

CHAPTER

3

The Method Up Close

DAILY LIFE for average people provides a limited opportunity for expressing the dynamic emotions and act-hunger that pervades their inner thoughts and feelings. They are generally locked in to specific daily rituals and expectations that they often find boring and dull. If the average person confronting the normal complex problems and issues of contemporary society had the possibility of a psychodrama session available to him once a week, he would be provided with the opportunities to dramatically live-out the many motivations that are now buried or suppressed and to resolve the many conflicts or dilemmas that affect most people's lives. A close analysis of the elements of psychodrama reveals how this form of expression would help you to act-out safely and to learn how—where necessary—to revamp your life performances for a fuller, more satisfying existence.

Psychodrama has considerable adaptability and flexibility. All that is required for a session is the conflict (philosophical or concrete), the group, and a psychodramatist. The freedom for a group to act out its problems is represented by the freedom of space on a stage, or any open space. (There are a variety of sessions that can be enacted without a trained psychodramatist present. These possibilities, with specific instructions, will be discussed more fully in the following chapters.)

All psychodrama sessions have several intrinsic elements: a *director*—the catalyst of the session; a *subject* or *protagonist*—the individual who presents a problem and represents the group in the session; the *auxiliary ego*(s)—who plays the role required by the protagonist for presenting the problem; and techniques such as *role-reversal*, the *double, mirror,* and the *soliloquy.*

The group present is crucial to a psychodrama because all members are considered participants. The group is not an audience as in a theatrical production. Many members will participate actively at some point in a session as auxiliary egos, but even those who sit through a session without speaking are expected to be empathetic and identify with the protagonist and the problems being presented. There is no place for critics, disinterested people, or voyeurs in the group, although sometimes their presence is unavoidable.

In contemporary practice, there are literally thousands of approaches to psychodrama, group process, and role-playing. Yet there is a classic type of psychodrama, and this will be the focus of the following descriptive analysis. A close comprehension of classic psychodrama provides the foundation for a therapist or group practicing psychodrama to move from the basic approach and become more innovative, spontaneous, and creative. Understanding the fundamentals of classic psychodrama and practicing them facilitate the creative adaptation of the method to a group's specific needs and to the effective use of psychodrama as an adjunct to another therapeutic modality.

There are generally three phases to a classic psychodrama session: The *warm-up,* which involves members of the group tuning-in to each other's concerns and focusing on a protagonist and a problem or series of problems. The *action-phase* is the heart of the session and involves the role-playing portrayal of various key scenes and the use of various techniques necessary to reveal the problem and move toward its solution. And finally there is the *post-discussion* phase, which involves an intensive examination by the protagonist and the group of the meaning of the session. In this phase the group at first, rather than being diagnostic and analytic, is expected to share with the protagonist emotional reactions which pertain to the session. For example, rather than saying to a young man who has just presented a session in which he acted-out his hostility towards his father, a man who in this case always squelched his freedom of expression, something analytic like "You really hate your mother and have displaced this aggression onto your father," it would be more appropriate to share your feelings about your own parents and honestly state how the session touched your own life. Even if an analystic or interpretative statement is accurate, at *first* it would be more appropriate for a member of the group to share his personal relationship as it related to the session.

It should be noted that not all responses or personal observations to a psychodrama in the post-discussion are uniform or follow the dominant group impression of the meaning of the session. For example, I recall a very intense and dramatic session with a young man in his twenties named Monroe. He was bedeviled by the constant and insidious intrusion of his mother into his life. In the various core scenarios he presented, she intruded into his life even into his twenties by telling him, among other things, in great nagging detail: how to dress, what to do at work, what he should or should not eat, the girl he should marry, etc. Even after he moved out of his mother's house, she would pull surprise white-glove inspections at his apartment and nag him about his cleanliness.

After about an hour and a half of Monroe's psychodramatic performance, he commented succinctly: "She has made me a complete and utter nervous wreck." This was evidenced by the fact that Monroe's body was shaking with rage from the onslaught of twenty years of subservience to his mother's every whim.

In order to give Monroe some respite from a draining session, I sat him next to me before the group and opened up the session for discussion. One elderly stoic lady in the group, who sat quietly through the session, seemed relatively unperturbed by Monroe's plight. (During the session, Monroe told me that she reminded him of his mother.) I asked the woman if she would be good enough to comment in this post-discussion by sharing her feelings about and reactions to Monroe's problem. She emited a long-suffering sigh and soulfully replied: "I know what that mother must have gone through with a son like that."

The feedback phase tends to enlarge the scope of discussion to include the entire group. At a later point, after group members have revealed their personal responses to a session, the director may encourage the group's feedback on valid analytic comments they might have noted in the protagonist's performance. In some cases, after an intensive action session, psychoanalytic, transactional analysis, primal, or Adlerian interpretations are welcome, if relevant. The main point is, however, that the analysis is appropriate only after action.

There are various kinds of warm-ups to a session. To open a session, the director might simply and directly ask, "Who would like a session?" Very often with a group that has been meeting regularly that is all that's necessary to launch the action. With other groups, more time in a warm-up may be necessary to help the group focus in on a relevant subject.

The director must be super-conscious of body language during the warm-up phase (and of course during the session). Some people who verbalize a desire to have a session may belie this motivation by their body posture. In contrast, I recall walking into the theater of psychodrama to direct a session and before I could say a word someone in the back of the room blurted out in a loud voice, "You'll never get me up there!" I looked at the man and noted his body seemed like a coiled spring. The only comment I made was, "Okay, come on up." With that he charged up on stage and moved directly into a very emotional problem. His pre-warm-up negativity was really a cry for help and a session.

Not all warm-ups are that rapid or spontaneous. For many groups it is advisable to lead in to a session in a more contrived or elaborate fashion. Another interesting warm-up for a group is referred to as "Lifeboat" or "The Survival Game." It parallels the 1940's film *Lifeboat*. The movie concerns a number of people in a lifeboat adrift at sea. The boat is sinking and everyone would certainly drown unless they put "the least valuable people" as determined by the group to its survival, one at a time, at regular intervals over the side. In the psychodramatic form of "Lifeboat," the session begins by having eight to ten members of the group volunteer to come forward and sit in a semicircle, as if they are in the lifeboat. The psychodrama director then briefly informs them of the premise of the role-playing situation. "You are in a lifeboat that is slowly sinking. In order to maximize the possible survival of most of the group, the group must vote every three minutes on putting a member over the side. In order to vote most judiciously in this situation, we will *first* have each member of the group take up to three minutes to state *why they should survive*." In a sense this rhetorical question raises the basic issue of the meaning of your life. In the many sessions I have run with this warm-up, the following summarized comments emerge as typical responses:

> "I should survive because of my children. They need me and I'm the best one to care for them."
> "I should survive because I'm the oldest one in the group. I have more wisdom to offer."
> "I should survive because I'm young and have my life before me."
> "I'm an artist and have a great deal of beauty to offer the world."

In other patterns of response, an attractive female seductively informed the men in the boat that they would not be sorry if they kept her alive. On another somewhat bizarre and humorous level, a young "Hollywood starlet" playing the lifeboat game bluntly stated, "I should survive because I'm the best cocksucker in

Hollywood." (Everyone laughed, but I noticed her answer clearly impressed several men in the "boat.") The "revolutionary" in the group usually suggests dumping the director and the game overboard (interestingly, this has never materialized); a group "lawyer" argues the rules; a person fearful of rejection sets himself up for an early vote overboard and protects his ego by telling the group to vote him out first, because he is the least useful member of the group. These are only a few of the varied responses. The most interesting aspect of this warm-up is that it forces a person to succinctly present his or her *reason for living,* and in the process the group rapidly moves to a deeper level of emotional communication.

The next phase of the role-playing game is the voting-out-of-the-boat process. Every three minutes the group votes someone out by secret written ballot that is tabulated by the director. The three-minute interval allows the group to interact by discussing their life, or asking other members of the group questions. As in life, if someone becomes too pushy, they may set up a negative vote against themselves. Also as occurs in the human situation, a person who is too eloquent or self-assured threatens the group, is defined as a "smart-ass," and is voted out for the wrong reasons. The person with the most votes after each interval is "out." (If there is a tie vote, all of the tied people are voted out.) It is interesting to watch the voting when it narrows down to the final three or two. In a triad there is the possibility of two people "making a deal." But this often backfires against the "dealer" and he is voted out. Often when two people are left, one (and sometimes both) will "suicidally" vote themselves out by indicating that the other person is worth more than they are. They can afford to be magnanimous because they have successfully "outlived" the rest of the group.

There are obviously many interactional intricacies and byplays that emerge in "Lifeboat," and it can be emotionally upsetting for some players. It is, however, a fascinating warm-up that rapidly moves people to encounter emotionally their reason for being.

More developed innovative warm-ups of this type include, for example, "the magic shop."

In the "magic shop" warm-up, the director may become the shopkeeper or he may appoint someone from the group. The shopkeeper opens by talking about the wares in the shop. "I have courage, love, longevity, beauty, freedom, sexual satisfaction, etc. And I will barter with you for any item you want." Someone in the group indicates they want more courage. The shopkeeper asks, "What are you willing to give for courage? It's a very valuable-salable item." The person offers cowardice, and the shopkeeper tells him, "We have stacks and stacks of cowardice. We give it away. Offer me something valuable." The "purchaser" says, "I will give you ten years of my life. I would rather live a shorter life than a life of compromise." The director zeros in and asks the potential protagonist how he compromises. Now the protagonist begins to talk about his life in the business world and how he has compromised his ideals and inner beliefs and become a "yes man" to his many bosses. The warm-up and the session thus move from the abstract to a concrete life dilemma. The magic shop is best utilized by having several people participating as purchasers, since the process tends to warm up the entire group.

The foregoing are more exotic and abstract warm-ups; the following is a more typical group warm-up. A group of about fifteen people enter the room and are seated. The director warms up the group by opening the discussion on feelings about occupational choice. One person says, "My main hang-up with work is that my mother wanted me to become a doctor and anything else I do is considered inferior. Somehow, underneath, I agree with her and anything I do seems second best and unsatisfying." Another group member says, "All bosses bug me. I just can't take orders from anyone because my father was such a dictator. I go nuts when someone tells me what to do."

As the discussion widens, the director notes that a number of group members express concerns with bosses as authority figures. He therefore selects an individual with an authority problem as a protagonist to represent the group's emotional mood on that day for that session.

An obvious first scene in the role-playing phase of the session would be to have the individual act out a scene with his father in which he was subjected as a child to what he considered to be outrageous orders and discipline. This type of session might involve the entire group in a discussion of the relationship between "work" and discipline in the family setting and work in an outside job.

Once the group has selected the area with which it will be concerned and has chosen the protagonist—that is, the person in whose personality the problem area is most clearly shown—the action phase begins. Essentially, what has happened is that we have established channels of communication through which the action on stage and the feelings of the group can merge into beneficial processes of catharsis, the development of insight, and relearning. Vicariously, the entire group tends to benefit from the action process through catharsis and the expansion of their perceptual fields.

As the protagonist is warmed-up to the roles that he is to play in relationship to the people who are causing difficulty in his current or past life, other members of the group are selected to portray the roles of people in his environment, or social atom. The protagonist may select an auxiliary ego on the basis of them looking the part. Sometimes auxiliary egos are selected on the basis of their own needs, or opportunities inherent in the situation for developing insight into themselves. For example, a young woman in the group has an alcoholic mother. A situation emerges in which I need someone to play an alcoholic mother. I would use the young woman in that role. In other words, the auxiliary ego chosen for a part may be someone for whom the experience of taking the particular role will be useful, although sometimes a person simply plays the role essentially for the benefit of the protagonist.

The following are further examples of using an auxiliary ego for the benefit of both the auxiliary ego and the protagonist. In a session with a young man who had a "drill sergeant" father, when a role of that order emerged in another person's session, he was cast in the severe father role to see what it felt like (to be like his father). In another session, a wife who felt she was constantly sexually beseiged by her "oversexed husband" was cast as an auxiliary ego in the role of the oversexed husband with a woman who had a similar problem. This enabled her to comprehend what it felt like to be the pursuer rather than the sexual object.

Psychodrama is primarily a group process, although it may shift from the group to focus on an individual's problem at varying points in a session. The director constantly moves toward mobilizing the group to work together on their problems. Even though one member of the group—the protagonist—serves as the session's focus, he functions as a focal point for communication within the entire group. Therefore, the production on the psychodrama stage represents an intensification and a more controlled extension of some of the problems of the total group. While action goes on, each person in the group participates through identification with individuals and emotional themes, extending these experiences in his own fantasy and often moving into the action as an auxiliary ego to the protagonist on stage.

The response of a member of the group not on stage is sometimes greater than that of the person on stage as the protagonist. The intensity of response to a psychodrama session, therefore, *does not exclusively* relate to a group member's participation on stage.

As an example of the therapeutic impact on a seemingly nonparticipating member of the "audience," I recall a young man who was a member of a group I ran for several months that focused on resolving family problems in a juvenile institutional setting. Over this period, he never said a word or moved on stage, yet I had the distinct feeling he was involved in all the sessions and in his own way benefiting from them. One day I decided to work more directly with him. I invited him to come on stage and introduce himself. He didn't respond in any way and was in an almost catatonic state. He was so withdrawn that he acted as if I were talking to someone else.

He was attired in a Navy pea coat, wore dark glasses, and hunched himself into a corner. His name was Bill, and after he resisted my invitation I began to talk *about him* as if he weren't there. "Who here knows Bill?" About four hands in the group of fifteen shot up in the air. "Has anyone here ever seen him under stress?" One young man, named Jerry, began to relate his observation of Bill on visiting day fighting and arguing with his mother (Bill hunched deeper into the collar of his pea coat). I asked Jerry to come forward and be Bill in combat with his mother. Using this *mirror technique,* Jerry as Bill began to denounce the woman playing Bill's mother. "You don't have any time for me—you never did. You love that pig [his stepfather] more than me. Why come around here acting like you care— you don't give a shit about me. No one does."

As Jerry mirrored Bill in the scene, the real Bill began to come to life. At first he took off his glasses, then his jacket. He began to breathe harder, identifying with Jerry-as-himself. He then moved forward into a chair closer to the stage. He began to react. When Jerry was *right* in his portrayal, he laughed and shouted, "Right on." When Jerry was wrong, he yelled to me, "No, man. That's bullshit. I never said that." Finally I said, "Why don't you go in and play yourself." By then he was very warmed up to his conflict with his mother and entered the session as himself. He had a fine, intensive session.

The session produced a number of insights about his dependency-hostility toward his mother, plus an improvement of his relationships within the group that was useful in later sessions with him and others. He also revealed, for the first time, *that even though he seldom talked, he had participated in his own way as a member of the group* in *every session.*

Growth and personal progress in psychodrama takes place through effective channeling of the group's dynamics for the benefit of its members. In a spontaneous group, which is free to express its underlying sociometric dynamics (the group's relationships), progress takes place *in situ* in the immediate situation. The role-test of the protagonist's growth and effectiveness in a problem situation happens in the session. Unlike discussion therapy, in which the client must now go out into the world to test his insight and growth, in psychodrama the improved performance of the protagonist takes place in the immediate session. In this sense, the session becomes a "screen test" for life.

A subject, for example, who acts out his problems through hostility is confronted with the consequences of his aggression on the spot, when the aggression can be dealt with by him and the entire group. A man who symbolically "punched" his wife in a psychodrama session (he had never actually done it in the reality of his everyday life, although he always wanted to) can see the size and shape of his hostility. We often get conflicting results. Some people who thought they had only a little hostility discover it is of super proportions when they punch a pillow (symbolizing the object of their venom). And some who felt they had powerful hostility discover it was minimal. Obviously, we do not want the protagonist to punch his wife in real life. Psychodrama, however, provides a safe, harmless opportunity to express long-suppressed feelings of aggression and, in some cases, guilt.

Emotions about parents are more complex than love and hate. *Guilt* is often a strong emotion. Many middle-aged people have child-ego states in which they feel they have "hurt" or "let down" their parents. The guilt emanating from these feelings often becomes the basic guiding theme in their problematic life.

One of the most extreme cases of guilt I have ever encountered in directing psychodrama involved a young man I will call Jerry. He appeared at a session one night when I was directing sessions in New York at the Moreno Institute back in the fifties. A common cultural theme session in those days involved a young Jewish male attempting to extricate himself from the tentacles of his overprotective mother, often by moving out of the house. The process inevitably was accompanied by enormous guilt for deserting his "Yiddishe Momma." (Yiddishe Momma has become a generic term for a smothering syndrome that goes beyond Jewish Mother. It applies equally to Italian, Irish, Polish, black, Chicano, and many other ethnic or racial mothers.)

At the time of his session, Jerry was about thirty and overwhelmed with guilt. The session, in essence, revealed a rather unique scenario. Jerry had been released the week before from a mental hospital after a two-year stay. He was hospitalized a week after two tragic events in his life: he was married and his mother died. The session, in summary, revolved around the following circumstances.

"The one thing my mother always stressed to me all my life—besides not eating in restaurants because 'all restaurant food is poison'—was that I should never marry a shicksa [a non-Jewish girl]. His mother always added to this "thou shalt not," "If you marry a shicksa, it will be the end of me."

A core flashback scene of the session involved Jerry in a phone booth with his new wife waiting outside as he phoned his mother about the event.

JERRY: Mom, I married a wonderful girl.
MOTHER: Tell me what I want to hear. . . . Is she Jewish?
JERRY: No, Mom, but I love her.
The phone clicks. In the next scene, Jerry visits his mother and reveals that not only was his bride Gentile, she was Eurasian.

Three days later Jerry's mother died of a heart attack—the exact end she predicted for herself if he married "out of the faith." Jerry became distraught with grief and guilt, linking his mother's death with his marriage. By further probing in the session there was no clear evidence in any direction that revealed a cause and effect link between Jerry's marriage and his mother's death. But no matter, because Jerry believed that this was the case. He had the marriage annulled and was hospitalized a week later with a "nervous breakdown."

As an attempt at assuaging Jerry's guilt, we had his psychodramatic mother tell him in many different ways that she died of a physical problem and that there was no emotional connection between his marriage and her death.

The overall and subsequent sessions had some positive effects of relieving Jerry of some of his guilt. He began to function reasonably well, but he never fully believed he was not guilty.

In summary, there are many complex dimensions to the powerful influence of emotions about parents. Some of these negative feelings can be adjusted through the group dynamics of the psychodramatic process. For those people who have pure love for their parents, it is simply not necessary or useful to have a session on this issue. But for the many relatively normal people who bear some hostility or guilt, it is useful to explore these emotions.

In my psychodramatic research in thousands of sessions, I have discovered that many people at some time in their lives (at times motivated by parent-induced guilt) have had the fantasy of killing a parent. They are often given this opportunity in psychodrama. It is a curious fact that many people have a precise idea of how and where they will do it, including the exact weapon they would use. In typical "psychodramas of parenticide," after the parent is symbolically killed we have the protagonist recite a eulogy over the deceased, as if at a funeral. The group members present become the mourners at the funeral. The eulogy usually reveals the protagonist's lifelong attitude and feelings toward his parent. The technique is useful since it reveals to many people at least three possibilities: (1) that they have a realistic view of the nature and intensity of their hostility; (2) that they underrated the degree of their venom; or (3) that they overrated their hostility. In most sessions the group psychodrama reveals the truer, deeper feelings that people have toward their parents— the basic socializing agents in their lives and the people most dominantly responsible for their identity and self. Following are the essential aspects of a psychodrama exercise on parental feelings.

Phase I. Each person in the group takes five to ten minutes to verbally express his feelings of love, hostility, or guilt for each of his parents. This serves to warm up the group to these feelings.

Phase II. The person who appears most warmed up to a session selects his director from the group and then presents several key scenes from his life that express the reason for his hostility or guilt.

Phase III. After he has expressed his negativity, he is supplied with an auxiliary ego parent who fulfills all of the ideal views he has about a loving, compassionate parent.

Phase IV. The protagonist reverses roles, becomes his real parent, and is asked questions that attempt to elicit the reasons why he or she has failed as a parent.

Phase V. In the post-discussion all of the members of the group talk about their personal-emotional points of identification and differences related to their parents and the protagonist's parent.

Basic Elements of Psychodrama

THE PROTAGONIST

The protagonist in a production tends to represent the group in his psychodramatic performance. He is the star of the session and his problems are presented. Before relevant action takes place, the protagonist must warm up to himself as he functions within the group setting, and this warm-up allows him to bring forth pertinent areas of concern and to exclude those areas that are not related to the concomitant group process. Some defenses and blocks he has used for years become so obviously superficial in psychodrama that for the first time it becomes possible for the protagonist to move spontaneously into deeper levels of his problem and to achieve a greater realization of himself. For example, many people maintain an idealistic-romantic notion of their marriage. Often, when they move into a session, their thin cover is blown and they reveal the depth of their discontent. Often, this revelation of the *real situation* of a husband and wife serves as the foundation for ultimately strengthening their marriage.

The protagonist, with the aid of auxiliary egos and methods such as role-reversal and the double, objectifies his problem in a situation. His perception of the situation—his "here and now" construction of it—is what counts, since this is the problem being worked out. What happened "in fact" in a past situation is not the immediate concern of the group or director at the time of psychodramatic action. The group and star are accepted on their levels of function, and an attempt is made to create a climate in which these levels of functions may be improved. For example, in session, if an individual is giving a portrait of someone known to the group or who might be present, and he is grossly distorting the other person's "real image," he has a license to do this because the session is involved with the protagonist's personalized perception of the situation.

As an example, in one session, a young man, Joe, portrayed his father as a combination of Hitler, Godzilla, Frankenstein's monster, and King Kong. The third session Joe brought his father to psychodrama. The group was amazed to see a 5'5" Mr. Milquetoast. But this in no way altered Joe's right to his perception of his father—in psychodrama. The awesome figure of *the person he psychologically perceived was real for him.* After a few sessions, however, he began to respond to his father more in accord with the reality of the nice man seen by the group.

The protagonist, in summary, sometimes for the first time in his life, is allowed to produce his unique emotional version of a person or a situation. During the session, he is the author of the scenario. Being allowed to present your perception of a phenomenon in itself is often a cathartic relief and has intrinsic therapeutic benefits.

For example, in a session with an obviously wealthy and beautiful lady who from the group's perspective "had everything," it was determined that her self-concept was that she felt poor and unattractive. The group, for several sessions, respected her version of her condition, which, briefly analyzed, related to her obviously low self-esteem. In later sessions the group was able to infuse her with their consensual reality of her condition. She would never have accepted this version of her real status at the outset.

The protagonist of a session, therefore, is allowed the freedom to sketch his own portrait of his life with limited interference. In some cases it is the first time that the person is in control and attention has been paid to his perception of life.

THE DIRECTOR

According to Moreno, the director "has three functions: producer, therapist and analyst. As producer he has to be on the alert to turn every clue which the subject offers into dramatic action, to make the line of production one with the life line of the subject, and never to let the production lose rapport with the group. As therapist attacking and shocking the subject is at times just as permissible as laughing and joking with him; at times he may become indirect and passive and for all practical purposes the session seems to be run by the patient. As analyst he may complement his own interpretation by responses coming from informants in the audience, husband, parents, children, friends or neighbors."

The director is the prime coordinator and *catalyst* of a session. With group input he determines who will be the protagonist and then orchestrates the flow of the session. The role of the director often fluctuates in the course of psychodrama sessions. His function is dictated by the demands of the situation at any given time. He may be passive or aggressive, kind and nurturing, or caustic and tough. The director may often double behind the protagonist or auxiliary egos, adding insights and commentary to these roles. At times he may become an authoritarian father or a demanding mother. There is no limit to the range of roles that may be demanded of the director. The only limits to the roles he may take are those set by the boundaries of his ability and the demands of the protagonist and the situation.

The director must constantly diagnose the situation within the group—including the action—and create new situations by means of which self-defeating patterns have maximal opportunity for being resolved. It is essential that the director have the ability to think on his feet and observe nonverbal as well as verbal communication cues in the protagonist and the group while carrying on his primary function of directing the session in such a manner that insight and learning is achieved.

In a sense the director is a field general and orchestrator of the session. He must not only be aware of the protagonist's emotional state but also must constantly survey the mood of members of the group. For example, on many occasions the protagonist is mildly into a scene and suddenly a member of the group who is more involved breaks into tears, or in a more subtle fashion sits tensely involved in the action. It is the director's role to be cognizant of these cues and responses in the entire group and to amalgamate these reactions into the overall psychodrama.

A psychodrama director, unlike a therapist in an individualized setting, is always subject to appraisal of his action by the group. The director is never excluded from the group's appraisal. In a psychodramatic atmosphere, he is not able to blame his difficulties with the group on transference or defensiveness by the protagonist. He is forced by the group to receive help from them in terms of recognizing that often a subject who accuses him of being overly hostile is quite right, and that this may bear little, some, or no relationship to the real authoritarian figure in the subject's life. A director must always be willing, in his relationship with the group, to allow criticism and to deal honestly with it when it develops. The psychodramatist, in addition to being a catalyst, participates in the group's action. He is at all times both a member of the group, as well as its leader.

AUXILIARY EGOS

Auxiliary egos are members of the group who are used as extensions of the director and the protagonist in the session. For example, a person who has "a controlling mother" in his head who is always directing his behavior, making his decisions as to what is proper or correct behavior, will in psychodrama confront this figure "in person" as an auxiliary ego. Someone will fill out and play the role of this mother so that the protagonist can confront this vector in his psychological monodrama.

The person—or the *image* of a significant person someone carries around in the monodrama of his psyche—may be real and accurate. In either case, confronting that *auxiliary* ego or image "live" in psychodrama is beneficial.

For example, in one session a young man presented an impotency problem he had with his wife. In brief, he had great difficulty gaining, or maintaining, an erection, and when he did he often had a premature ejaculation.

It was learned in the early scene of his session that he had, like Jerry, what he termed "a domineering momma." She had warned him all during his early life that if he married someone she disapproved of that it would hasten her demise. Partly because he was rebellious, and partly because he fell in love, he committed the atrocious sin of marrying a beautiful girl whose religion and social status were wholly unacceptable to the mother.

My therapeutic hypothesis was that the image of a disapproving momma, who produced enormous guilt in the man, was present in bed with him and his forbidden wife. When confronted verbally with the possibility that his guilt about defying his mother's basic edict produced his impotency, he commented, "Although my mother hasn't died from my relationship so far, it's entirely possible that my mother is responsible for killing my hard-on."

In a core scene, I placed the young man in bed with his wife, played by a female auxiliary ego. They simulated foreplay. In the psychodrama he actually acquired an erection as they lay together on the floor of the stage (although he joked about it). I then sent in an auxiliary ego to play his mother. She physically got between him and his wife in bed and said, "Here you are in bed with this lower-class tramp. What have you done to me? I can't hold up my head in the neighborhood. You'll never be happy with this girl. You shouldn't mix up the blood. God forbid you should have a child with her!"

Obviously, the young man's mother was never physically in bed with him and his wife. Psychologically, however, he acknowledged that the auxiliary ego mother's statement was very close to some of his deeper feelings of guilt when he went to bed with his wife, and when the auxiliary mother made her poisonous statements his erection went down.

In the scene we had him physically throw his "mother" out of bed. He ferociously carried out this suggestion, returned to his "wife" in the psychodrama bed, and said, "I really love you, and I'm never again going to let that bitch intrude in our marriage. We'll never even visit her again or let her come to our house unless she behaves herself."

In subsequent sessions the young man psychodramatically entered into other aspects of the triangle of himself, his mother, and his wife. As the underlying problems of his relationship to his mother became resolved, the sexual and other aspects of his relationship to his wife improved. Several months later he informed the group that he no longer had the symptom of his former problem and that his sexual relationship with his wife was now vibrant and satisfying.

The injection of an auxiliary ego in a session facilitates production and intensifies the meaningfulness of interpersonal situations. Auxiliaries may enlarge or exaggerate the scope of the roles they play in order to help the subject examine more dimensions of his problem. The group setting in general, plus the use of auxiliaries, allows a great diffusion of transference phenomena. The great range of personalities available for interaction that is supplied by auxiliaries results in a more rapid development of total involvement in the therapeutic setting of the group. This is especially true of auxiliaries who take the part of significant figures in the life of the subject and of group members whose behavior reflects prototypes of familial figures. This spread of transference phenomena affords greater mobility, and greater objectivity, than occurs in individual settings or other approaches.

Auxiliary egos sometimes are trained professional personnel. In some situations, such as working with an extremely regressed, hospitalized patient group, this type of auxiliary is necessary. However, in a group that embodies the range of normal human problems, regular group members usually function quite well as auxiliaries.

Usually, the auxiliary ego functions on a spontaneous level, responding to the demands of the situation within the group. There are some situations in which the auxiliary ego role may be highly defined. For instance, if the director wishes to test one of his hypotheses concerning a particular subject's ability to function when confronted with a specific kind of problem pertinent to his life, the director may coach the auxiliary. The director may coach the auxiliary, "Go in and play a husband who wants a divorce" to test the possibility in a session. Or in a heated argument between husband and wife, I often send someone in as an auxiliary ego to represent the couple's children so that they can assay the impact of their battles on the children.

Auxiliaries taken from the group are often given specific role assignments pertinent to their own problems. For example, an auxiliary ego having a problem with his own parent may develop an understanding of his problem by taking the role of a parent in a session portraying someone else's problem.

An auxiliary ego may not only be a person. He can be a concept or symbol—such as God or the devil—an inanimate object—such as a person's house, a creative product of art—or whatever is required to help the protagonist present his problem. A religious person, for example, might pray to his unique God, in a session and get a response from an auxiliary ego who portrays *that* God. An auxiliary ego can also portray an inanimate concept such as "wealth" or an artistic object. In one session an artist talked to his "painting" as played by an auxiliary ego; in another a writer talked to his "best book" and expressed his emotions about it.

The auxiliary ego, in brief, plays the vital person or component required by a protagonist to enact his problem of conflict in a significant situation. The person who becomes an auxiliary ego must be flexible enough to fulfill the protagonist's needs in a session. A good auxiliary ego responds sensitively to the nuances of the protagonists' emotion and aids him in objectifying his internal vision of his emotional world.

Specific Methods and Techniques

There are numerous psychodramatic production techniques used in sessions to aid the protagonist and group to achieve states of spontaneity and creativity. These are techniques employed to bring about a maximum of creativity, productivity, and growth in a session. Psychodramatic production techniques have evolved from the experiences of many years. Techniques are applied in the course of the production at the moment when they seem indicated and are usually not planned in advance. It is essential that the director be sensitive to the group production so that his use of these techniques sparks the production, lends support, and produces insight for the protagonist and other members of the group. Timing in the application of techniques is of crucial importance. Following are some of the basic techniques used in psychodrama and the rationale for their use.

ROLE REVERSAL

Role reversal is the procedure in which A becomes B and B becomes A. For example, in a mother-daughter session, a protagonist who is the daughter may reverse roles with her "mother" (an auxiliary ego) when indicated in the situation. Roles are reversed for a number of reasons.

1. A protagonist, when playing the role of the relevant other (e.g., the daughter becomes her mother), may begin to feel and understand the other person's position and reactions in the situation. This may enhance the protagonist's "telic" sensitivity (two-way empathy). The daughter learns more about how it is to be a mother to herself as daughter.
2. Role reversal may be used to help the protagonist see himself as if in a mirror. The daughter playing the role of mother will see herself through her mother's perception. This instrument has the effect of producing insights for better understanding by the protagonist as she sees herself through the eyes of a significant other. For example, a daughter who reversed roles with her mother better understood her mother's motivation. She commented, "From the vantage point of my mother, I saw for the first time that she feels badly about her age and her looks and is putting me down—because she has begun to compete with me."
3. Role reversal is often effective in augmenting the spontaneity of the protagonist by shifting him out of defenses. In a typical

case a protagonist engaged in the same "fight" with a spouse for years. Each adversary had played the same role in a tired script with no solution. The role reversal will often shake up and change the form that the conflict takes and produce new insights. Part of the learning is that the role reversal helps the protagonist to understand others in the situation through being them.

4. Role reversal is often used simply to help an auxiliary ego to better understand how a role is perceived by a protagonist. The auxiliary, although not having been on the actual scene of a situation, attempts to fulfill the requirements as projected by the subject. For example, in a mother-daughter interchange in which the real daughter is the only one present and there is an auxiliary ego playng the mother, if the daughter plays her mother she cues the auxiliary ego into how the role should be played. The subject, therefore, who is usually the only person who has experienced the situation, will take the role of the other, through role reversal, so that the auxiliary may more effectively fulfill the role as the protagonist sees it. This enables the protagonist and auxiliary to move more effectively into the problem situation, at least as it is perceived by the protagonist.

In general, the role reversal has the effect of taking a person out of himself so that he can get a look at himself from the "others'" point of view. Some people initially are very effective at taking the role of another; others require considerable spontaneity training before they can meaningfully reverse roles. Still another aspect of role reversal is the fact that protagonists can play certain "other roles" in their life very well and some ineffectually.

For example, I recall having a woman in a session reverse roles with her husband, a man to whom she had been married for fifteen years. In the role of her husband, I asked her to soliloquize *his* thoughts. After five or ten awkward minutes, it became apparent that she had a limited idea of what her husband thought or even said. In the session she manifested a pattern of nonstop talking at her husband. She seldom had any empathy or awareness of his position or emotions. This was precisely the problem with their marriage. After the role reversal, the husband, who was in the group, breathed a sigh of relief that at last the group and even his wife could see the problem. She was given the "psychodramatic prescription" of reversing roles in their day-to-day lives when they would get into states of conflict. The role reversal became a remarkable vehicle for improved communication between the husband and wife, and their marriage prospered.

Another remarkable example of role reversal took place in a session I ran with an outpatient group at a state mental hospital. A member of the group, Jim, a man of about forty, requested a session because of a problem he had with getting employment. He had some complex personal problems, but a dominant surface symptom that no doubt blocked his chances for employment was the manifestation of a nervous body tic and a slight stutter in his speech. When he was nervous, his face would twitch, his body would periodically, involuntarily twist around in a slight convulsion, and he had a slight stutter. A check of his medical record revealed that there was no marked physiological-neural problem and that the doctors felt his tic was psychosomatic.

Jim came up on stage and we proceeded with a session in which he sought employment in a factory as an assembler. An auxiliary ego played his potential employer.

EMPLOYER: Tell me about your work history.

JIM: Well, I worked for ten years at the X Company. Then I had some personal problems and I was hospitalized for a year. Now I'm fine and ready for work again.

As Jim spoke in the interview, his body and face were nervously twitching and he stuttered.

L.Y.: Okay, Jim, reverse roles. Play the role of the potential employer.

Jim left his self-role as a twitching, nervous, potential employee. *Remarkably, as soon as he reversed roles and became the employer, his body became completely calm, with no sign of a twitch, and he spoke clearly without the slightest stutter.* Jim's awareness that in other roles he had control over his involuntary body movement and his speech helped him immensely in reducing his nervousness. He was finally successful in acquiring a reasonable job.

The role reversal is an excellent technique for getting out of oneself for a time and perceiving one's identity from another vantage point. Empathy, or taking the role of another, is at the center of all human interaction and communication. The process of physically and emotionally doing this in psychodrama enhances more accurate self-other perceptions and facilitates more meaningful communication.

THE DOUBLE

In the double experience, the double attempts to actually *become* the protagonist. If the protagonist is A, the double is A. The double sits close to the protagonist and physically and emotionally tries to assume the protagonist's posture. The double adds a significant dimension to the protagonist's performance. The protagonist is instructed by the director to respond to his double. For example, a protagonist may be expressing love, and the double senses that the love is real but is also covering up hate. When the double expresses a feeling of hatred, at the same time the protagonist is expressing love, the protagonist has several alternative responses to his double: (1) if, the double is right, he can simply agree with the double's statement; (2) the protagonist can disagree with the double and vehemently state his love with such great anger that the group suspects the validity of his protest ("Methinks he doth protest too much"); (3) the protagonist can ignore the double's comment; or (4) the protagonist can disagree in a manner that reveals this disagreement is an authentic feeling.

The protagonist's response to the expressions of his double is revealing and generally useful to the session. The double enhances the protagonist's action and often adds dimension to his performance. A double is used to enlarge a situation in order to help the protagonist's performance. When the protagonist is honestly and effectively presenting his point of view, a double is not necessary and may in some case negatively interfere with the protagonist's action. When used properly, a double gives a protagonist much needed support. For example, in a session with a young man who felt oppressed by his father, the double helped the son gain the courage to talk back to his overwhelming father for the first time.

The double can help a protagonist express feelings of fear, hostility, or love that he is unable to verbalize on his own.

The director of a session may determine that a protagonist is frozen or role-bound in a scenario. After a few moments of interaction in which the same lines are repeated between the protagonist and his relevant other, the director may have the double carry on with the same repetitive accusations and recriminations. The director may have the protagonist step aside and watch as an observer or as in a mirror the scene from his stale script.

The double may also take a chance and express certain hypotheses that are hinted at in a situation. For example, a double may say to the protagonist's boss, "I hate you because you're just like my father." The protagonist may confirm or deny the double's statement. The protagonist may or may not agree with many thoughts the double expresses. Is this respect, the double is useful in helping the protagonist produce new cues or lines of further understanding. The double produces added dimension to the protagonist's performance that he, for various reasons, cannot present himself.

I can recall in one session my wife, Donna, doubling for a lady who was having a session in which she encountered various serial lovers, whom she found dull and unsatisfying. The lady was attired primly and properly in, as I recall, a dress with a lacy Peter Pan collar that gave her a cute-little-girl look. But when she began to act psychodramatically, her overt appearance of arch-primness cloaked her more basic perceptions of men who displeased her, especially her husband. I recall her opening line to the auxiliary ego who played her husband: "You're okay, but you're much too hairy, and your prick is too short." The rest of her diatribe against her husband and other men was in a similar vein. No one, apparently, according to her portrayal, could properly satisfy her enormous sexual appetite.

In the session she portrayed herself as a super sexually liberated woman who found all of "her men" mundane. In the center of one interaction, her double, for no special reason, based on what the protagonist said but derived from a feeling as her double, exclaimed, "My problem is that I've never had an orgasm." The protagonist wheeled around to her double, broke into tears, and with amazement said, "How did you know?" The double thus propelled the protagonist into a more honest portraiture and broke past the false image the subject was trying to project. She began to reveal that beneath her sexual bragadoccio, she was a frightened little girl who was really afraid of men and sex. Often, a double in a role will have an insight that is not apparent to anyone in the group, including the director, and this will open up the protagonist to his deeper, more honest feelings.

In addition to helping to break through to deeper feelings, the double tends to become the protagonist's friend and helpmate in difficult situations, often providing the necessary support that enables a protagonist to master complex and difficult situations in psychodrama and that facilitates successful behavior later on in his life.

THE SOLILOQUY

The soliloquy is a technique that parallels, as one example, Hamlet's soliloquy in Shakespeare's play. It involves the subject reciting his thoughts out loud in the middle of a scene. It is a useful technique for expressing the hidden thoughts and action tendencies of the protagonist to himself and the group. The protagonist's soliloquy is often parallel to his overt actions. For example, a person overtly expressing love and affection may be feeling love and affection. At other times, however, a person expressing love overtly may be feeling subjective hatred, and this will be expressed in the soliloquy. It is important to have the protagonist express both emotions, and the soliloquy aids in this process.

The soliloquy in most respects parallels the process of "free association" in psychoanalysis, with one significant difference: in psychodrama the soliloquy is performed in the contextual fiber of an *actual situation*. Also in psychodrama, as differentiated from psychoanalysis, the process is utilized not only for analytic purposes but also to facilitate the dramatic action of the session.

The double technique may be combined with the soliloquy, in which case the double may soliloquize for the protagonist in a crucial scene.

I recall a session with a man who was having sexual problems with his wife. In brief, the husband and wife had become bored with each other's sexual performance. In the simulated psychodrama that he enacted with a female auxiliary ego who played his wife, the man was having intercourse with his wife. Overtly, as he was having intercourse, he made extravagant declarations of ardor and love. His double began to soliloquize what he felt were the man's covert thoughts. The protagonist soon joined his double in a synchronized soliloquy. "I wish she could come—I want to get it over with. I'm hungry. I wonder what's in the refrigerator. Did we finish that whole roast beef dinner? Is there any left over?, etc." The wife, who was present in the group, remarked, "I know when he's just stabbing me or making love. And if he's off on a trip, I just viciously hold onto him, resist my orgasm, and let him suffer as long as I can."

After several sessions, the husband and wife obtained a deeper understanding of each other's motives and feelings and became more honest and attuned to each other's moods. This resulted in greater feelings of affection and their relationship improved, including their sex life.

The unstated soliloquy is a part of every human interaction in everyday life. Many times a person's inner thoughts relate closely to the overt spoken words, but too often—particularly in crisis or problem relationships—there is a disparity between what people say out loud and what they think underneath. The soliloquy in psychodrama is a useful tool for bringing these hidden thoughts to the surface. Soliloquized thoughts are vital to understanding conflict and resolving human problems.

FUTURE-PROJECTION TECHNIQUE

This method involves having the subject act out, with the support of auxiliary egos and a group, a meaningful situation in which the subject expects to act in the future. The effectiveness of this procedure depends on the significance and importance of the situation for the protagonist and the extent to which the auxiliary egos are able to actually project the protagonist into the future. It is also important that the protagonist *really* is going to participate in the situation in the future at a given time. An intense, effective warm-up is the essence of the application of this method. As many particulars and specifics of the situation as possible should be emphasized in the warm-up.

This method, like other psychodramatic approaches, rests on the solid foundation that an individual's thought level can be acted out with the help of a group. The "future" is often most detailed on the thought level. For example, I recall a session using this technique in which a protagonist exclaimed, "He didn't say that" about a situation that he had never lived out. This indicated that he was psychodramatically presenting a situation that was not new to him. It had been "acted out" many times on his thought level. However, psychodramatically the action, with its many added dimensions, was more vivid and productive for the subject through the aid of the method and the group.

The future-projection technique can prepare a protagonist to perform more effectively in a future situation. I recall another psychodramatic session in which the protagonist, a young married man, revealed how he separated from his wife. They had experienced a violent argument three months prior over some complex differences, and had been separated for that period of time. He was, at the time of the session, scheduled to meet with her and his son the following week to discuss either a reconcilation or a divorce. He was understandably quite anxious about the event because he was unsure of his feelings and had to make a decision about their relationship.

In the session, he warmed up to the situation by first describing the plane as it came in from where he stood at the airport. Then, with the help of a double, he soliloquized what he was thinking while waiting. It was determined through a soliloquy that he had not decided whether to act "nice" or "nasty" toward her and that he was unsure about continuing the marriage. He also felt that "she has probably poisoned my son's mind against me" and did not know how his son would act toward him.

He then psychodramatically met his wife and child as portrayed by auxiliary egos. The egos fulfilled his precise conception of how they would act. This was accomplished through having the protagonist reverse roles with his "son" and "wife" and act out his view of how they felt about him. It was a very emotional production, since the protagonist had already lived through this situation many times on his "thought level." When he "met" them psychodramatically, he broke into tears.

With the help of the group and the auxiliaries, the subject explored several possible future-oriented alternatives: his wife wanted a divorce; she was glad to see him and sorry she had left; she was indifferent; his son ignored him; his son was glad to see him; his son was full of misconceptions about him. In the session, as he reviewed all of these possibilities, he began to sort out his own feelings about what he wanted to do.

His tension about the future-scene was reduced. As he expressed it: "I now have a much clearer picture of what I can expect and I don't feel as worried as I was." He also felt that he had learned a great deal more about how he "really" felt about his wife. After the session, he felt that he really loved her and wanted to try to "start all over again," whereas before the session he was unsure on this point.

In talking with the subject the following week after the real meeting, he remarked that he felt much more sure of himself and was able to communicate this to his wife, who was quite tense. He felt that his clarification of the situation produced by the future-projection technique helped him and his wife get through a most difficult period in their relationship. Because of the psychodrama future-projection, he felt peculiarly familiar with the *real* scene and was consequently in better control of himself and the situation.

The future-projection technique helps the subject to articulate for himself his objectives in a real situation. In the psychodrama many dimensions of the situation will emerge that the subject never considered before on the thought level. In the same vein, it helps him to clarify his role within the situation in relation to others. He may discover that he is anxious about the forthcoming situation because he really loves (or hates) the other, or has feelings he had not previously considered.

The future-projection technique is a *preparation* for an important life situation that will aid the subject in presenting himself most effectively and honestly; at the same time, it enables him to be helpful to the other individual(s) involved. The group is invaluable in the future-projection technique and can, if properly warmed up, share with the subject similar experiences that they had encountered as an aid to the subject's preparation. The group members will know the life situation better, since they have "been there" before psychodramatically.

If properly administered, the future-projection technique can be most useful in a wide range of possible future situations: from one loaded with emotional intensity and anxiety, e.g., the man who had a meeting scheduled with his former wife, to a simpler situation involving a conference with a potential employer. When applying the future-projection technique, it is important to bear in mind the necessity of producing an intense warm-up and the fact that the psychodramatic action may very well influence the protagonists behavior in the real life situation.

In one session I ran, the protagonist, Rod, had contemplated leaving his wife and getting a divorce for several years in his monologue. He had been married at that point for twenty years. In the session he admitted that he had thought about it over and over, and that it now obsessed all of his thoughts. He further stated that he had never admitted this possibility to anyone before. In brief, his session, which finally involved the future projection technique, took the following form:

Scene I. Rod acts out his basic conflict with his wife and decides to leave her.

Scene II. He goes to a divorce lawyer. As the complicated emotional aspects of the divorce settlement are hammered out, we note that Rod becomes more and more emotionally shaken.

Scene III. He is in a depressing motel room he has selected ("It's all I can afford"). He sits depressed, paces, doesn't know anyone to call, feels lonely.

At this point in the session, Rod tells the group, "You know what I want to do now, I want to get the hell out of here. I don't want psychodrama, analysis, or anything. I want to go home!"

Rod left the group early. The following week he reported how he rushed home, kissed his surprised wife as he came through the door, and then hugged each of his children. "We had a great dinner and I never enjoyed being with my family more," he said.

The session and the future-projection technique gave Rod an opportunity to explore the possibility of separation and divorce. After experiencing these possibilities psychodramatically without, in fact, causing his family the pain that would have resulted if he had actually left, he determined that he really didn't want to break up his family. Of course, he had problems with his wife that required resolution, but after the psychodrama experience he was extremely motivated to work on them in order to keep his marriage together.

THE MIRROR TECHNIQUE

In the mirror technique, an auxiliary ego portrays someone who is reluctant or unable to perform for himself. The mirror involves a stand-in for the protagonist. Often when a protagonist sees someone "mirror" his performance, he comments: "Do I really act like that?" If the auxiliary has done a credible job, the group will chorus affirmation. The mirror enables a person to examine his performance in a significant situation from sufficient distance to gain some perspective and insight on his behavior.

The mirror effect thus enables a protagonist to see for himself how he acts in a situation of relevance. The mirror is used whenever it is indicated that it would be productive for the protagonist to see himself in action, as if in a psychological mirror. It helps withdrawn subjects warm up to self-presentation as, for example, in the cited case of the young man in the juvenile institution.

The protagonist is always encouraged to comment on, or react to, the auxiliary therapist playing the mirror role. At times the protagonist will participate, come forward, and take over his own role from the auxiliary when he is sufficiently warmed up. In this context he has an opportunity to alter his performance in a more effective direction.

Methods and techniques are only aids for helping to produce therapeutic production and interaction in psychodrama. They are never ends in themselves. They are only available means, and may be sensitively adapted to the process and produce benefits for the protagonist and the group.

A skillful director may use these methods in a productive way to facilitate the diagnosis and solution of the protagonist's and the group's problem. When utilized by a talented director with the aid of sensitive auxiliary egos from the group, these techniques and methods become part of the natural flow of a session. In this sense, the director becomes an artist in the cause of a productive psychodramatic performance.

CREATING NEW METHODS

Technique and method are adapted as the group dictates; they do not dictate to the group. An unskilled director may use methods arbitrarily that are not closely related to the protagonist's and the group's needs. An axiom of psychodrama is to do what helps the protagonist and the group most. It is a psychodramatic principle that what helps most are those techniques which facilitate spontaneous action and a testing of realistic alternative solutions to a problem. In the course of these trials, insight into the dynamics of the structures of the groups are sharpened and broadened. A psychodramatist is frequently challenged to produce, on the spot, new methods and techniques to meet the needs of the group and the protagonist.

I recall, for example, a session with a young man and his wife who were concerned about his impotency problem. Specifically, he had difficulty gaining and maintaining an erection. The group member had previously had a medical examination which revealed that his basic problem was emotional and not physiological. After several exploratory psychodramas that produced no change in the couple's situation, we finally had a breakthrough.

In the successful session, on the spot I conceived the idea of having a trained auxiliary play the role of the man's penis. The crucial scene in the three-hour session involved the man and his wife (played by a female auxiliary) and took place in their bedroom. The auxiliary ego, as "the penis," was placed between them. (The real wife was in the group.)

HUSBAND: Let's make love, darling. You're so beautiful.
(Auxiliary ego penis begins to sag.)
WIFE: I want to, but I refuse to be left frustrated again!
(Auxiliary ego penis begins to sag further.)
WIFE (*caustically*): How much can I take of this. Look, you're getting soft again.
(Auxiliary ego penis starts slumping to the floor.)
HUSBAND: Well, let me give you some head. Maybe it will be okay again.
WIFE: No, I don't want any excuses. If you can't do it the *right way,* forget it.
(Penis slumps and lies flat on floor.)

The group and the protagonist laugh a bit about the serious way in which the auxiliary ego plays the penis. This nervous laughter tends to relieve some of the pressure of the session.

The scene was replayed. This time the auxiliary ego "wife" was supportive and agreed to any sexual activity that made her husband happy. She also assured him that an erection was not necessary, that his mere physical presence turned her on. The real wife in the group noted the modification of performance.

During this supportive and cooperative replay by "the wife," the auxiliary ego penis stood ramrod straight. The wife and the husband broke through into a discussion of their more basic interpersonal hostility and moved toward resolution of their mutual sexual problem.

The group reinforced the obvious analysis (from their own experience) of the immediate situation: that the man could not perform in part because of the restricted expectations of his wife. His wife's *only* criterion for successful performance was an erection. When the husband could relax and was given the right to "fail," and some of the couple's more basic interpersonal problems were resolved, the situation took place in a session that removed the blockades of hostility the spouses felt for each other. When these were removed, they no longer felt the need to punish each other in their love-making performance.

The *creative* use of an auxiliary ego penis served several purposes. It highlighted the problem as it related to the couple's interaction. It also gave a painful-grim situation a touch of humor, which opened up the protagonists and the group to some different ideas.

There are a variety of less bizarre innovative devices that have emerged in psychodrama. In fact, all of the now standard methods (role-reversal, double, mirror, soliloquy) were once innovations that aided in the production of a session.

A more standard yet innovative approach each time it is used is the *psychodrama of dreams*. The exploration of a dream in psychodrama involves a creative director, since dreams, unlike the scenarios of day-to-day life, can become quite surrealistic. Despite this, following the protagonist's lead, the session attempts to articulate the substance of the dream.

The warm-up to the dream session should start with the protagonist going through his or her ritual in going to bed. Positioning is important: Do they dominantly sleep on their back, front, or side? If they are sleeping with another person, which side of the bed are they on? How are they dressed, or are they undressed?

After the protagonist is "asleep," the director should let the first sequence in the dream emerge spontaneously. As in one case, the protagonist may begin: "I am in a room in a strange house. I am

seated at a table eating with a group of strangers. People are talking, but it's like lip sync, without sound. . . ." At about this point,
I had the protagonist set up the room in her dream (color of walls,
books in bookcases, type of drapes, etc.). She then set up the table
and chairs and selected four people from the group who as closely
as possible fit the description of the relatively nondescript people
in her dream. She then sat at her place at the table and began
to soliloquize further into the dream.

In this case it rapidly became apparent to the protagonist
and the group that her dream masked her repressed bitterness
about the vacuous quality of her family life. The scene was in
actuality the situation between her, her husband, and her two children at the dinner table. "We all talk but there is no sound . . . ,"
no real communication.

In most dream psychodramas, there is an element of protagonist hypnosis. The colors and lights, positioning of people, or
specters of things are important. In some cases, as in the foregoing
example, the meaning of the dream becomes explicit; in others,
interpretation is required. After a dream sequence, it is extremely
valuable that members of the group share their own dreams in
the post-discussion phase of the session.

A dream sequence that was fairly explicit had the elements of
what I would term a preventive psychodrama. A young lady begins to talk about a recurring dream involving her husband. (He
was present at the group session.) She comes forward and begins to
act out the dream. In the dream sequence, she enters a room and
finds her husband in bed with another woman. "I don't see them
balling, but I know they've made it." She gets furious with both of
them, since her husband and the other woman in the dream
vigorously deny what she sees.

Her dream usually ended with her waking up distraught. She
then enacted how the dream was so real. She would then begin in
her awakened state to chastise her husband. The dream had occurred around five times in a two-month period. The husband in
the session turned to the group and implored, "How the hell do

you deal with this kind of accusation? She's driving me nuts!" The wife agrees she's behaving irrationally, but she can't help herself.

In the session, we next moved into an actual psychodrama scene that had occurred five years in the past, when the husband *had* a mistress. The circumstances of the wife (as the protagonist) finding out and confronting her husband were enacted. The husband in the group squirmed and sweated throughout the session and had one interesting reaction to the replay of his past peccadillo: "She has a remarkable memory."

In summary, the husband denied that he was being unfaithful at that time—the dream was never repeated—but the wife felt she was experiencing all sorts of subtle cues that her married life was repeating itself. In a *later* session, the husband admitted that she was right. "I was really shook up at your dream psychodrama because it was so close to the truth of what I was doing." In later sessions, they explored the reasons for his and her discontent and worked out some reasonable solutions. The dream psychodrama had opened up a facet of their relationship that had been suppressed in reality.

In addition to the basic methods of psychodrama, new devices and techniques, such as dream sessions, bringing to life inanimate objects, producing and objectifying fantasies, are all useful in the production of a person's scenario. A creative director best accomplishes this type of production by faithfully and artistically following the protagonist's perceptions of the world and maximally utilizing the intelligence of the group present at the session.

Significant Aspects of the Psychodrama Method

An awareness of the group's structure or its sociometry is fundamental knowledge to a psychodramatist in directing a session. Sociometry, briefly defined, refers to the network of relationships of a group. For an individual person, his sociometry is his social atom, or the significant relationship in his life. Everyone is at the center of a web of relationships that have importance to them, and this comprises their social atom.

In psychodrama the group and the individual are simultaneously the focus of the therapeutic process. Their inextricable relationship is considered at all points in practice. Although one or the other may be the focal point of activity at a particular time in a session, the psychodramatic director is aware of his responsibility to both the individual and his social atom.

The psychodramatists's guiding principle is that, to help resolve problems, the focus must be on the sociometric network of relationships, as well as on the individual's personality dynamics, which are hinged to his social atom. Awareness of the group's dynamics and the behavior manifestations of underlying sociometric and personal difficulties is an intrinsic part of sociometric understanding. It is necessary to understand the individual's social atom in order to understand him and his particular problems. Part of psychodrama therapy is to help the individual to understand his own unique social atom—his structure of primary interpersonal relations.

When working with the specific problems of any member of the group, the director recognized varying involvements on the part of the whole group and utilizes the group's sociometry, in the therapeutic process. This may be done through interpretation and particular role assignments for group members taking auxiliary ego roles.

A subject is entitled to be the star of his session. When it appears, however, that a member of the group monopolizes the protagonist role in session after session, the director must be aware of this phenomenon and modify it to give others an equal opportunity.

The skilled psychodramatist will continuously assess the group's sociometric structure for maximum rehabilitation objectives for all the members of the group. The director shifts emphasis according to his perception of the group's need, gained through his interaction with the group members as they create their productions. This determination of effectiveness is made through sociometric procedure. Psychodrama thus is an approach that has a diagnostic method built into the operation. The director continuously assesses the group's structure through sociometric analysis, and this enables him to determine moves that are of maximum benefit to all people in the group.

Psychodramatic sessions produce scenes that approximate the problem-producing everyday setting more closely than any other form or approach. Immediate problems, born of the group's interaction, are dealt with *in situ*. These are extended to situations that exist with significant people outside of the group, and by the use of auxiliary egos and various production techniques the opportunity is afforded for corrective emotional experiences to occur. Defeatist, repetitive patterns can be seen and treated more readily. Perhaps more important, distortions in perception of interpersonal relationships become recognized, and attempts are made to achieve more realistic views on the spot. Group members often express valuable insights and interpretations and form new relationships with each other. All of these patterns enhance the resolution of problems.

The subject or group discover they can handle a problem in reality after they find they have done it psychodramatically. Psychodrama comes closer to the "life-line" of human experiences than perhaps any other therapeutic format for the simple reason that it is lived out more intensively and extensively than the stresses of living would permit on the outside. The psychodramatic world is given characteristics of "surplus reality."

In intensive psychodrama, the emphasis is placed on aiding each person to develop a realization of himself, in all of his roles, in a setting in which errors of judgment and behavior are not so traumatic as they would be outside of the therapeutic setting. Every attempt is made to work toward an expanded and integrated self-perception, with its concomitant attributes of interest in others and concern, not with the existence of problems, but with the ability to deal with them—in other words, to work toward being a freer and more spontaneous person. Acting in the theatrical sense is not the focus of psychodrama. The goals are to aid in self-realization rather than to promote the development of actional facades.

The spontaneous subject pulls the group with him into the light of sociometric experience and understanding. A new light is thrown upon symbolic behavior on the psychodramatic level of action because it surpasses and encompasses life. In action, body language or nonverbal communicative patterns become apparent, and maximal use may be made of them: movements, postures, gestures, facial expressions, pauses, and body attitudes often tend to indicate the more fundamental feeling tone of the protagonist than his words do. Conflicting feelings are clearly stated when nonverbal communication shows internal consistency, or when verbal and nonverbal communication are at variance.

The time factor is another significant variable in psychodrama. Although a production may be focusing on past, present, or future, psychodrama is always in the *"here and now."* The subject is his current conception of a situation. The problem that is objectified with the aid of the group and auxiliary egos is what is troubling the subject at this time. It may refer to similar conflicts in the past, and to similar potential ones that may appear in the future. If the conflict becomes clarified and understood, the subject and group can experience their handling it effectively in the immediate session. If they cannot handle it to their satisfaction, the action may be repeated until the anxiety and conflict of the problem is reduced or resolved.

Reality testing and evaluation takes place on the spot within the session itself. The subjects learn to live and to communicate directly. Psychodramatic experience indicates that when a subject has not resolved an issue or conflict satisfactorily, the difficulty will reappear in the following psychodramatic session. However, when he has worked out the problem, it becomes apparent in the group session; proof is already visible in the psychodrama. For example, progress in relating to a spouse, feelings about one's level of "success," and other issues may be clearly observed in the session. Later, reality testing in the actual situation will usually validate the individual's progress in the "practice" setting of his psychodrama group.

In part, therefore, psychodrama is a rehearsal for life. In a session, a person can experiment with many modes of performances. He is neither time-bound nor role-bound and can reach out creatively into a number of variations on new spontaneous themes of life. He can explore the supernatural, death, relating to his God, or any other circumstance he, the director, or the group feels would be productive. And the acting-out, unlike daily life, is nonpunitive. Psychodrama thus provides an opportunity to explore one's existence in this widest array of possibilities. Although in certain respects psychodrama is a rehearsal for life, it must be remembered that acting-out in psychodrama is also a bona fide existential experience that affects the protagonist and the group in a fundamental way. In this regard, psychodrama is per se a life experience that has validity and meaning apart from its beneficial impact on life.

CHAPTER

4

Psychodrama and Other Therapies

IN THE PRACTICE of classic psychodrama, most practitioners creatively utilize some facet of almost every other relevant therapeutic system. In psychodrama we have observed and used primal responses to help unblock basic pain emanating from early life repressions; in a Gestalt manner, we have used empty chairs to represent relevant others in a person's life (with role reversals); in post discussions of sessions, we have used psychoanalytic concepts (e.g., ego defense mechanisms, unconscious motivation, etc.) to account more systematically and perceptively for behavioral patterns; in some sessions, the basic conceptual scheme of biofeedback has been utilized (for example, in one case to unblock the psychosomatic problems of a hearing block). *In brief, psychodrama in its foundation and evolution has been eclectic in attempting to use any or all concepts that help people to reduce psychic pain, obtain greater insight, enlarge their perspectives on life, and enhance their life performances.*

In the same manner that psychodrama has been nurtured by other systems, many other therapeutic modalities can benefit from psychodramatic concepts and techniques. The introduction and usage of psychodrama in other therapeutic approaches has already occurred in a spontaneous fashion. Several specific cases make this point: Fritz Perls acknowledged that Gestalt therapy was in large measure derived from psychodrama; in Transactional Analysis, ego states of *parent, adult,* and *child* are often enacted in a psychodramatic fashion; a number of neo-Freudian psychoanalysts have patients act in psychodrama and then interpret the action in classical psychoanalytic terms; many of the principles and techniques of Dr. William Glasser's Reality Therapy overlap with psychodrama; psychodrama has been fundamental to the encounter approach since its inception and has been widely utilized in various *sensitivity and encounter groups.*

A comprehensive coverage of psychodrama as a possible adjunct to *all* other therapeutic modalities would go beyond the scope of this analysis. It is useful, however, to further detail the relationship of psychodrama to a variety of significant therapeutic modalities with some specific suggestions and guides to the uses of psychodrama as an adjunct. From this didactic analysis I am hopeful that professionals and laymen in the practice of various treatment systems—including those not specifically discussed here—can interpret ways in which to creatively and usefully integrate psychodrama into their approaches.

In the following analysis, I will discuss and analyze psychodrama in relationship to and as an adjunct of general private practice, discussion and encounter group therapies, Synanon, Gestalt therapy, primal therapy, Transactional Analysis, and reality therapy. In a final segment, I will discuss the utilization of psychodramatic techniques in the classroom situation for resolving emotional problems, improving the transmission of information and knowledge, improving the students' intellectual ability, and dealing with the complex social issues that have become part of the educational system.

Psychodrama as an Adjunct to Private Practice

Many effective individual therapists have spontaneously incorporated psychodrama into their practice; others have been more directly influenced by psychodrama as a consequence of participation in a session. The following example is prototypical of many experiences that have been reported to me by therapists who have participated in classic psychodrama and then used psychodrama as an adjunct to their private practice.

A psychiatrist engaged in individual therapy who had attended a psychodrama I directed called me several days after the session and with great excitement related "a breakthrough experience" he had with a patient after he used the psychodrama technique of auxiliary ego for the first time in his practice. I recalled his spontaneous participation in the session: as an auxiliary ego, he had dramatically and insightfully played the role of a protagonist's father. His psychiatric orientation was essentially neo-Freudian, and he was open to and eclectic about the use of other techniques. The following is a summary of his verbal report to me on the use of psychodrama in his private practice.

The patient I used psychodrama with was Joe. Briefly, he is handsome, forty, a playboy type, who claims to want a permanent relationship with a woman but flits from woman to woman, constantly complaining about the emptiness of his transient bedmates. Of course his problem on a deeper level is a basic hostility toward women emanating from his unresolved relationship and hostility toward his domineering mother. His fear of getting involved with one woman causes him to pick women—who have enough faults from his viewpoint—so he can easily eliminate them if it gets serious. In my three years of therapy with Joe he raged and sometimes cried about all of the things his mother has done to him—both because he believed she did not love him and because she never gave him any approval, no matter how successful he is as a lawyer. The last year of his therapy has been a broken record on these themes.

The psychiatrist's therapy with Joe had been stalled over the past year and he dreaded meeting him because the sessions had become a complete bore. The therapist felt guilty about his negativity toward Joe, yet when Joe appeared he was confronted with a deadly dull fifty minutes; and, more than that, he couldn't think of any new emotional territory to cover that would help Joe. The patient would present the same problem with slight variations, and the therapist would offer the same tired analysis about him and his mother. After participating in my psychodrama as an auxiliary ego father, the therapist decided to try some role-playing with Joe.

When Joe came in, he launched into a tirade about an upsetting phone conversation with his mother in which she picked on everything he was doing and called him "a bum with women": "Why don't you get married and give me a grandchild?" and "You work too hard and don't get paid enough." All of these comments, Joe told me, reduced a forty-year-old man to a blubbering five-year-old screaming back at his mother.

The therapist described the psychodrama he had participated in and then asked Joe if he would be willing to try a different approach to his problem. After he explained psychodrama in more detail, Joe agreed and they role-played the fight he had had with his mother over the phone, with the therapist playing his mother.

I was amazed how fast Joe got into the scene. I must have played Momma perfectly because rather rapidly he was screaming and crying at me, about how I (as his mother) didn't love him, never wanted him, and didn't appreciate him as a person. I also held up a pillow, as I had seen it done in your session, and let him hit it. Believe me, he pounded it as a symbol of his mother for a full five minutes.

In the middle of playing his mother, several new thoughts occurred to me. The main one was that I was a lonely, morose widow and the way I held onto my son was to badger him. This kept him guilty and angry yet involved with me. In the role of Joe's mother in the session, I made this point and several others.

Another thought that struck me in the role of Joe's mother was that I withheld any approval of my son because my disapproval seemed part of the magnetic force that held him near me.

In our post-discussion of the role-playing, Joe said he felt better because it was the first time he could say anything he wanted to his mother. I, of course, did not restrict his language. Also he had never in his life hit his mother—but he felt that pounding her in the form of a pillow was a real catharsis.

Anyway, the session was a huge success in that it opened up new emotional territory and also the time we spent together, since the role-playing has been more interesting and productive.

A bond of greater closeness between Joe and me has developed since our session. He told me that because of the session, especially the way I played his mother, he really believed for the first time in three years that I understood him and his problems. The one session broke up our frozen situation and provided fuel for a number of productive sessions in my usual mode of practice.

Another pattern of psychodrama in private practice has involved my running sessions of classic psychodrama with patients—*with* their therapist present. In fact, in most sessions I have directed in clinics or hospitals, I insist on having the patient's therapist present. Several psychiatrists who have participated in this type of arrangement have reported that the psychodrama tends to generate enough material for several sessions of productive interaction in private practice.

The described case of the therapist who used psychodrama in private practice marks a considerable advance from the practice of the classic form of psychoanalysis. Moreno, in one of his lectures, caustically characterized the gap between classic psychoanalysis and psychodrama in confronting some of the realities of the therapeutic situation:

> . . . the psychoanalytic situation was so modelled that it permits analysis and excludes action. The patient was placed on a couch in a passive, reclining position; the analyst placed himself in back of the patient so as not to see him and avoid interaction. The situation was hermetically closed; no other person was permitted to enter it and the thoughts which emerged on the couch were to remain the secret of the chamber. It was to omit the positive and direct relationship of the therapist to the patient. The technique of free association is not natural talk. The patient reports what is going through his mind. The transference of the

patient upon the analyst was not permitted to extend and become a real, two-way encounter. The conclusion is that the unconscious motivation behind the model is a fear on the part of the analyst of being put in the position of acting out towards the patient and being acted upon by him. It is a safety device against overt love and overt aggression. The difficulty is, of course, that by this, life itself was banned from the chamber, and the treatment process became a form of shadow-boxing.

There is a growing movement to utilize the best elements of individual therapy and psychodrama in private practice. The amalgam of processes does, however, require a better understanding of some complexities that deserve closer analysis—and some suggestions that will enhance the therapeutic process.

In some cases, the therapist might effectively employ another person to be used as an auxiliary ego in order to maintain the autonomy and purity of his therapeutic role. If the therapist feels more comfortable in this posture, he can use a psychologically oriented receptionist or secretary to help as an auxiliary ego. Some properly motivated assistants can play a variety of both male and female auxiliary ego roles. If the therapist does not choose to use an assistant and plays all of the roles himself, he should be aware of one significant complication: the patient, especially after an intense session, may have a degree of role confusion about the therapist because he will, in part, see him in the role he played (e.g., mother, father, spouse). There is a hypnotic quality in a deep psychodrama, and the protagonist can often lock the auxiliary ego into the particular role he or she has played.

As an example of this fixation on an auxiliary ego in a role, I recall a session at an institution for teenagers when a young man had an intense session about his mother. The young man, a client in the institution who played the protagonist's mother, cornered me the following week when I returned for another session: "Will you get Jim off my back? The punk thinks I'm his mother and he's been following me around all week long bugging me." Obviously, a client can deeply cathect and after a psychodrama continue to relate to a person in the auxiliary role he or she has played in a session. The individual therapist, therefore, who uses psychodrama in private practice and plays several hate-love roles—such as parent, spouse, child, even God—should be aware that this can produce a complicated role relationship with the patient, one in which his dominant role as therapist may be obfuscated or confused.

There are ways of overcoming this possible complication. It is best illustrated by my use of psychodrama on a particular occasion in private practice.

A young man was referred to me by the father of his former wife. For various practical reasons, I agreed to meet with him alone, rather than in a psychodrama group. The problem, summarized, was that he had been separated and divorced from his former wife for over five years. They had no children. He lived miserably in California and she lived happily in New York. He made a unilateral decision, often blocking out considerable negative evidence about his former marriage, that he really still loved his wife and that they should move back together. I knew from direct contact that the ex-wife was happy to be rid of him and had no desire to even see him again. This was corroborated by the ex-wife's father, who had tried on two occasions to dispatch the unrequited lover from New York back to California, where he had his home and a good job.

Although the man had deeper problems, my job in the one session I agreed to have with him was clear-cut: to convince him that there was no possibility of reconciliation. No words or actions by either his father-in-law or the object of his obsession, who hung the phone up on him over ten times, seemed to swerve him from his amorous pursuit.

When we met in the theater at the Moreno Institute in New York, we first sat on the stage and discussed the situation. It quickly became apparent to me that any hint of the stark reality of the rejection produced a furious, hysterical reaction. I briefed him on psychodrama and then I began to play the various auxiliary ego roles, first the role of his father-in-law and then that of his ex-wife. He responded with deep emotions.

One of the most important aspects of the session was my physical positioning of the several roles. The protagonist sat in one chair, and I set up three additional chairs for the roles of father-in-law, ex-wife, and myself. He quickly learned and accepted that when I was in a specific chair I was either the ex-wife, the father-in-law, or Dr. Yablonsky. The central point is that if I had stayed as I did, in the beginning of the session, in one seat or position playing these separate roles, he would have been confused.

Moreover, I noted that as his ex-wife, when I faced him directly (at first) he *did not hear* my rejection. I then sat in a chair behind him and played her as only a voice. When he finally began to relate to my rejection of him (as the ex-wife), I enlarged on my reasons, presenting explanations I had actually learned from his former wife. Finally, I faced him directly as the wife and clearly told him my negative feelings about him. He finally responded that he regretted the decision, but ultimately had no choice but to accept the verdict. The session was a success in terms of its limited goal. The possibility of role-confusion exists when the therapist plays all of the necessary roles in one physical position. This can be overcome, however, by positioning yourself appropriately. Move out from behind your desk—if you use one—and use specific seats for specific roles. When you return to your seat, this will signal the client that you are returning to your role as therapist.

PSYCHODRAMA AND TRANSFERENCE

On a deeper, more complex level, a consequence of incorporating psychodrama into private practice is its effect on the "transference" implications of the patient-therapist relationship. In Freudian terms, in its simplest form, transference refers to the process of transferring emotional attitudes and fantasies that a patient has toward a real person, who is part of his problem, onto his therapist. For example, a patient whose problem relates to father-hatred may transfer some of this hostility onto his therapist. In the Freudian theoretical context, transference is considered a useful process for the therapy. For example, the therapist can point out at an appropriate point in the therapy how the patient's hostility functions, and how some of the patient's hostile feelings have been transferred.

Psychodramatists have a somewhat different perspective on transference, in part because, in a group, transference energy is displaced onto various members of the group. There is no argument about the displaced aggression of transference on the part of the patient, but psychoanalytic theory does not adequately account for an equally important event: the therapist's emotional feelings about the patient. Strict Freudians almost deny the presence of what might be termed *countertransference*. In fact, as Moreno has pointed out, transference and countertransference are rather inadequate concepts for describing what actually takes place in individual therapy. Moreno uses the concept of *tele,* which, briefly stated, refers to the two-way flow of emotions between therapist and patient. The tele concept involves all attractions and repulsions between people in interpersonal relationships. It is the sum total of the emotional aspects of a relationship.

The concept of tele should not be confused with the related concepts of "empathy" and "transference." Empathy is an essential component of tele and may be defined as a one-way feeling into the private world of another person. This is the method by which we intuit the moods of others. Empathy, in effect, involves putting yourself in the other person's shoes. By its very one-way nature, empathy differs from tele, which represents the total effect each person has on the other. Putting yourself in another person's position not only helps you see things from where he stands but can also provide the potential for a change in your mood, producing the reciprocal emotional effect of tele.

It is a fallacy of some individual therapy that transference or the one-way flow of emotions of the patient should be emphasized without accounting for the tele effect. Psychodrama sessions often revolve around the circumstances of a patient in individual therapy who wants to explore his feelings about his therapist. In a session I directed, a patient encountered his therapist and his feelings of hostility toward him. The following is a key excerpt from the session that relates to the issue of transference.

Patient: I am really mad at you. I've been sitting here and we've rapped back and forth for a whole year. At forty dollars a session, I've paid you over $2,000 and I feel I haven't received any help at all.

At this point I had the protagonist reverse roles and play the role of his therapist to get the therapist's actual response.

Therapist (played by protagonist): We're finally making progress. You have transferred the hostility you have toward your father onto me. This is a real breakthrough. Now we can move ahead with your treatment. Let me explain transference to you. (A lengthy explanation of the meaning of transference is delivered by the patient in the role of therapist.)

When I shifted the protagonist back to his own role, he commented that this was his current dilemma in therapy. Was his negativity about his therapist and his failure an accurate observation, or was the therapist right in his analysis that "transference" was now a facet of their relationship? This, of course, was a vital area of discussion that needed to be brought back into his sessions with his therapist. My "psychodramatic prescription" to the patient was that in his next session with his therapist he should report his psychodrama session in detail. This two-way flow between psychodrama and individual therapy can facilitate therapeutic progress in both methodologies, despite the fact that in some aspects there is a difference of opinion and logic.

BREAKING UP A THERAPEUTIC LOG-JAM

At the most minimal beneficial level, the use of role-playing in private practice can (as in the example given) productively shake up an interaction that has become routine and unproductive. There are periods in every dyadic relationship in which people become locked into a rote-repetitive unproductive association. This condition can obviously also occur between a patient and a therapist. In this regard, a psychodramatic production can often produce new material and open up wider vistas for productive exploration.

In some cases, after a time, it is not unusual for an underground negative unconscious contract to develop between a therapist and a patient that blockades progress. This situation can develop when the patient presents a "token insight" into his problem that the therapist may accept because to probe deeper requires harder work in an uncomfortable situation. For example, the patient explains his behavior: "My acting-out is displaced aggression against my father." Whenever the patient "acts out," the therapeutic interaction is not pursued beyond the "displaced aggression against father" hypothesis. This type of negative contract enables the therapist to rest on his oars, and the patient can avoid exploring other parts of his psyche that might force him to confront his pain. The insertion of some role-playing into the patient-therapist relationship tends to shake up such negative contracts and helps to break new ground.

ONE PSYCHODRAMA PICTURE AND A THOUSAND WORDS

Incorporating psychodrama into other therapeutic situations can enlarge both the therapist's and the patient's perspective on a problem through moving from talk to action. As an example, a family therapist reported to me the productive use of role-playing in one aspect of a husband and wife problem. The new dimension provided a rich and valuable insight that led to the resolution of the couple's sexual problem.

Over a number of sessions, the husband complained bitterly in the family therapy situation about the fact that his wife rejected him sexually. She defended her rejection of him on the grounds that he approached her in a clumsy fashion. The resolution of their problem foundered on the words that were exchanged in the therapeutic sessions. A breakthrough occurred when the therapist, in desperation after hearing the same argument over and over again, had the couple role-play a typical approach-rejection scene portraying what took place in their bedroom the evening before. Several specific problems that had not been expressed in the prior verbalization became apparent in the psychodrama. Among them was the wife's soliloquy about the husband's approach as he acted it out in front of the therapist. "He is nibbling on my ear—he must have seen it in some rotten movie. It turns me off rather than on . . . I hate his cheap cologne . . . , etc." Although most of the comments were superficial, when they were spoken in the context of the situation they graphically illustrated the problem.

In another case, a counselor told me about a patient whose description of how he applied for a job bore little resemblance to his observation of the absurd way the client went at it—as expressed in a role-playing situation.

In a similar context, I recall a session I directed with a group of inmates at Riker's Island Prison in New York. The sessions were largely group discussions set up for inmates about to be released back into the community. The discussions were focused on potential problems related to release. One crucial issue discussed was acquiring a job. Each individual talked about how he was going to get a job, and then I had them role-play the situation of applying for a job. It was fascinating to watch some of the enormous disparities between the protagonists' verbal picture of a situation and their role-playing performance. In prison parlance, some "talked the talk but couldn't walk the walk."

One role-player, in particular, represented himself effectively on a verbal level, but was by his demeanor outrageous, insolent, and hostile to a potential employer in his role-playing session. All of his peers commented on his negative attitude and demeanor. He then replayed the situation more effectively in psychodrama and later on the outside, where it really counted.

It is useful in therapy to have a client role-play several key arguments or conflicts he has depicted to the therapist in words. The role-playing will almost always visually and dramatically reveal some valuable new information and often can provide key insights that are therapeutically productive.

Psychodrama and Group Psychotherapy

Psychodrama is, of course, a special form of group psychotherapy. Psychodrama is by no means only role-playing. In any classic psychodrama session, a considerable amount of time is spent in verbal group interaction. Specifically, the post-discussion phase of a session is essentially discussion group therapy.

Over the past thirty years, many forms of group therapy have proliferated on the general therapeutic scene. At first, many group therapy programs were essentially developed for the economic reason of one therapist reaching many patients. But increasingly, as therapists have become aware of the additional therapeutic benefits and implications of working with a group rather than an individual, the movement has grown enormously.

In recent years, many essentially individual therapists have begun to use group therapy as part of their practice. Some therapeutic modalities (e.g., Gestalt, Transactional Analysis, reality therapy) utilize both individual and group approaches. A variety of generic forms of group therapy—including encounter therapy groups, sensitivity training, guided group interaction, so-called T. groups, and consciousness-raising groups—have emerged. All of these tend to incorporate several parallel concepts into their methodology.

1. A contract is formed designating the goals of the group as well as the ground rules. The contract is either decided upon before the group is formed or formed by the group in its first meetings.
2. Open, truth-telling self-disclosure is considered a basic step toward growth and is generally insisted upon.
3. Confrontation is an important growth variable in the group. Confrontations attempt to explore human potentialities. They may be used to find the strength and weakness of an individual as well as to motivate a person into action. There are many types or methods of confrontation but they all have the same basic goal: to derive information that is either known or unknown to the self.

4. Even in encounter groups, provisions are made for supportive behavior. Participants are encouraged to learn how to react to the more dramatic dimensions of others and in a sense become co-therapists to each other.

5. The fact that most people in the same society are generally "in the same boat" emotionally is considered an important attribute of all group therapy. There is a tendency for people to feel better about themselves when they realize that others are encountering problems that parallel their own. This *mutuality* is a valuable factor in group therapy.

6. It is recognized in most group therapies that the role of group leader as therapist is modified. Except in severely autocratic group therapy approaches, the leader becomes more of a catalyst and the members of the group become co-therapists to each other. Further transference as a therapeutic concept is somewhat vitiated since "transference" is spread among more people and group tele is likely to be a more perceptive concept. Also the *effectiveness* of the therapist is clearer than in individual therapy. One person may be transferring negative judgments about the therapist, but in group therapy the consensual evaluation of the therapist is less likely to be the emotional distortion of transference; it is more apt to be a *realistic judgment* of the therapist and his therapeutic ability.

It is apparent that all of the factors described are also part of the psychodramatic process as group therapy. The added ingredient in psychodrama is the particular phase of a session when appropriate role-playing is utilized.

All group therapy can be aided by some adjunctive use of role-playing. There are natural occasions that emerge when a role-playing segment almost happens on its own. For example, a man has talked and interacted for a considerable amount of time about his marriage. An obvious move at the right time would be to have a woman in the group become an auxiliary ego and play his wife.

Also in group discussion therapy, the flow of the session can be enhanced by a variety of psychodramatic techniques, especially actual role-reversal between members of the group. Tom should become Mary, Jack should become Joe, and vice versa. In some instances, when members of the group feel they have something to contribute, they should "double" for a person of the "hot seat" in a session.

A standard exercise that can be employed is having different members of the group reverse roles with the group leader. This once occurred spontaneously in a group I directed that was set up as an encounter group. I arrived late one day to find a member of the group in my chair. He was a better impressionist than Rich Little; he invited me to be seated and began the session with himself as protagonist. What he, in fact, did was reverse roles with me. His exaggeration of my approach was a sardonic lesson about my "good-guy" pompousness. I was depicted as a benevolent despot. The lesson was bitter, but useful. As a result of my productive experience, I recommend that a therapist who is a hearty and secure soul periodically psychodramatically reverse roles with each of his clients. It is a useful experience for both parties, especially for the therapist.

In brief, the judicious use of psychodramatic methods in discussion group psychotherapy is recommended. A flexible group therapist who appropriately blends such techniques as role-reversal, doubling, and soliloquy into the flow of general group interaction can effectively improve the potency of the group sessions.

SYNANON *

Synanon is a social movement and approach to life that has helped thousands of people overcome a past of crime and drug addiction. In recent years, many people who were never addicts or criminals have benefitted from playing the "synanon game"— the organization's form of group therapy. Hundreds of imitations of Synanon have emerged in the U.S. and Europe. This pattern of expansion has had the effect of enormously enlarging the scope, impact, and meaning of the original Synanon organization. The movement was founded in 1958 by Charles E. Dederich, a layman

* For a more comprehensive discussion of synanon see L. Yablonsky, *Synanon: The Tunnel Back* (New York: Macmillan, 1965 and Penguin, 1967).

with a genius for understanding and solving human problems. The synanon game, invented and developed by Dederich, is the vehicle that drives the wheels of the overall organization.

In its basic form, about three times a week each member of Synanon participates in a synanon game with ten to fifteen people. The groups proceed to different parts of the house. Everyone in the group settles down, as comfortably as possible, in a circle, facing one another. There is usually a brief silence, a scanning appraisal of who is present, a kind of sizing one another up, and then the group launches into an intensive emotional discussion of personal and group problems. A key point of the sessions is an emphasis on extreme, uncompromising candor about one another.

The synanon game is, in some respects, an emotional battlefield. Here an individual's delusions, distorted self-images, and negative behavior are attacked again and again. The verbal-attack method involves exaggerated statements, ridicule, and analogy. In some respects, this "surplus reality" is a form of psychodrama. Attack therapy in a synanon game has the effect of "toughening up" a person. It helps him to see himself as relevant others do. He gains information and insights into his problems.

Synanon group sessions operate within a social scheme and under a set of conditions different from those of standard professional group therapy. The sessions are administered by a group of peers who have similar problems. Because of a similarity of life experiences and identifications, a fellow Synanist is more likely to be acceptable as a "therapist" than the usual professional. Also, compared with a professional therapist, the Synanist is *not* seen as an *authority figure* in the usual sense. Synanists can and do psychodramatically reverse roles as "patient" and "therapist" in synanon game sessions. The Synanist who plays the role of a therapeutic agent in a game expects, and often obtains, some insights into his own problems in the process of helping the other person. He often projects his own problems into the situation. This kind of cooperative therapy facilitates the realization of a true total therapeutic community, a live demonstration of Moreno's concept of the *total* therapeutic community, where everyone is a therapist (and at the same time a patient) to everyone else, as in psychodrama. Synanon involves a democratic approach to "psychological interaction." There is an absence of the usual status differences between "patients" and "doctors." This condition of equality among group members seems to facilitate a deep intensity and involvement. The emotional growth of each person in Synanon is of concern to everyone in the group. Everyone's success and personal growth is part of Synanon's overall development. An enlightened self-interest in helping the other member is a significant motivating force for all participants. In psychodramatic terms, as Moreno has postulated: "A truly therapeutic method can have no less an objective than the totality of Mankind."

During my research in producing a book on Synanon, I introduced psychodrama into the situation in several ways. At various points in time, with the aid of Charles Dederich, we had several series of classic psychodramas with select groups. In the process, I led special psychodrama sessions focused on specific issues. My research psychodramas included:

1. The meaning of drugs to an addict. For example, in several sessions we had ex-addicts talk to an auxiliary ego playing his drug. (I have also used this technique with alcoholics who talk to their liquor; this technique amplifies the meaning of the sedation to their emotional needs.)
2. Sessions on male-female relationships and marriage in Synanon.
3. Sessions on parents and the socialization of children in Synanon.

Since the organization's inception, founder Dederich has creatively developed the synanon game process. One innovation was the use of games in marathon sessions such as a "48-hour trip." Psychodrama techniques spontaneously became a part of "the trip," since toward the end of the trip, when people were most emotionally open, they often would spontaneously slip into a psychodramatic experience. In one trip I was on, a young man who had been raging about his "cruel father" for thirty hours of verbal group encounter sessions suddenly burst into tears about "Why didn't you love me, Dad?—I loved you." An intuitive person sitting near the young man (a person with no prior psychodrama experience) spontaneously began to role-play his father. The young man began to embrace his father, and the complex emotions of a lifetime began to spill out of him. As a result of episodes of this sort, the psychodramatic approach later was specifically built into the Synanon trip. As in other discussion group therapy, psychodrama is often a natural development in synanon games. For example, it is a natural progression when someone is raging about someone emotionally close to him to have someone play the role of the other. This can be built right into the fiber of the group interaction.

The leader of a synanon game (or a sensitivity or encounter group) who uses psychodrama should be aware of a fundamental issue related to physical and emotional positioning. When a person is on the "hot seat," as in a synanon game or encounter group, they are physically facing their "helpful" antagonists. In this face-to-face position, they can more effectively counterattack or defend their emotional posture on an issue. When the session veers into role-playing, the subject is *off guard from the group* and more involved in his personal emotional scene. Someone in the group should act as a psychodrama director during the role-playing segment to shield and defend the protagonist from any unwarranted or harmful attack from another member of the group.

When the person comes out of his role-playing session, any severe attack can be emotionally damaging because he is too vulnerable. Coming out of a psychodrama is like surfacing from a deep-sea emotional dive or emerging from a dark theater—it takes some time to get used to the group-light. The leader of the session should help the protagonist move out of his psychodrama posture back to his more defended position, where he is face to face with every other member of the group.

GESTALT THERAPY *

Fritz Perls, the acknowledged leader of the Gestalt therapy movement, expressed several basic guiding themes that were at the foundation of the Gestalt approach. One was that there was a continuing battle between fascism and humanism in most societies. He negatively reflected that most therapies attempted to make the patient "adjust" to society. He felt that the use of Gestalt therapy was a counterattack to a trend toward personal subjugation because it encouraged the client to become "real"—to develop himself in his own terms. This theme of humanistic people vs. the robot is, of course, the foundation of the psychodrama movement as explicated by Moreno in his early works. In Perls' Gestalt terms, the process of helping a client become "real" did not involve "analysis" or "adjustment" but the integration of personality.

Perls describes a person's ego boundary as the differentiation between self and otherness. In disowning a part of his self, a person shrinks his ego boundary; and the more parts of the self he disowns, the less energy and power he has. A central avowed purpose of Gestalt therapy is to fill what Perls referred to as the "holes in the personality," to take back such disowned parts and integrate them in order to become whole again.

For Perls, the process of growth involves the transference from environmental support (first from the mother, later from other adults, and finally from any manipulation of the environment to fill our needs) to *self support,* and meeting our own needs.

A basic goal of Gestalt therapy, therefore, is to make the transition from environmental support to self support, and Perls believes this is achievable by going through "the impasse." The impasse is the crucial point in growth when environmental support is not forthcoming but self support has not yet been achieved. Without the frustration of the impasse, there would be no reason to discover that you might be able to do something on your own

* This subject is explicated in more comprehensive detail in Fritz Perls' *Gestalt Therapy Verbatim* (Lafayette, Calif.: Real People Press, 1969).

rather than manipulating the environment in order to achieve it. Often, according to Perls, the impasse will turn out to be a fantasy, a catastrophic projection that keeps the patient from growing. Perls believes that the therapist acts, in part, as a projection screen (a modified auxiliary ego) for the patient and attempts to bring the patient face to face with his own blocks and inhibitions, "his way of avoiding being a whole person." In Gestalt therapy, self-awareness alone is the means for personal growth. "Awareness per se—by and of itself—can be curative," says Perls.

In this classic gestalt, the patient sits with the therapist on a kind of stage where he "works," and this work is not necessarily done before a group. When there is a group in gestalt, it sometimes functions as a kind of sounding board, in a feedback session after the patient has "worked." As in the psychodramatic post-discussion, the group's feedback is injected to give the patient some awareness of how he comes across to others. A psychodramatic session is similar, but a most significant difference is that in Gestalt *the group* is in most instances considered more important to the treatment than the therapist. In fact, the therapist-director in psychodrama is essentially a catalyst with some equality in group status; the Gestalt therapist is considered to be more of a supreme commander of the proceedings. In the psychodrama, after members of the group have taken roles as auxiliary egos, they are often more closely tuned in to the person's emotions than is the director. This does not happen in a Gestalt session. Only one person works at a time and usually only in a one-to-one relationship with the therapist. There are no auxiliary egos; the patient talks with relevant others who are represented by empty chairs. The protagonist may also reverse roles with an empty chair, a method also used in psychodrama.

A significant Gestalt concept is "the here and now." The patient is forced to analyze his motivations: How do I keep myself from doing something? How do I frustrate myself? How do I give myself pain? In the patient's awareness of his own process, according to Perls, lies the cure. The "here and now" in psycho-dramatic terms is not rooted as Gestalt to the present conflict alone, as it is in Gestalt. The psychodramatic "here and now" is a broader concept that recognizes the social psychological principle that all present thought and behavior is also rooted in past and future conceptions of life. The director in a psychodramatic session, therefore, is not necessarily completely obligated to the immediate situation. He may vary the session to the past, present, or future depending on the protagonist's perceived need.

In psychodrama the director also has a responsibility to the group that is not as evident in Gestalt therapy. ("The Gestalt therapist assumes responsibility only for himself.") A psycho-drama director produces a session in such a way as to fill the needs of both the protagonist and the group. The psychodrama director assumes a more directive approach than the Gestalt therapist. He suggests techniques, shares his own emotional experiences, and takes the lead in setting up scenes for a protagonist that he believes will be beneficial to the client's self-awareness and growth. In contrast, the Gestalt therapist is more likely to wait and see what "the patient will project onto his screen."

In both the Gestalt and the psychodramatic session, a drama is enacted. In psychodrama it will take place on the broad stage of life, whereas in a Gestalt session, it will take place in the "hot seat" on stage. The hot seat is the place "to work," an ordinary chair in which the patient will sit; by taking his place in this chair, he accepts that he is ready "to work."

The elements of psychodrama, of course, include role-playing, role reversal, doubling, and auxiliary egos. Similar elements are often used in Gestalt therapy, but with one important difference. The roles in Gestalt are *not* played by other persons. They are *all* played by the patient, since they are all seen as personal projections of the patient.

Role reversal used in Gestalt is similar to the psychodramatic technique of the auxiliary ego role reversal, but rather than picking members of the group to act as auxiliary egos, the Gestalt patient is given an empty chair. In that empty chair sits, in fantasy, anyone with whom the patient desires an interpersonal encounter. The empty chair may be a mother, a father, a husband, or a lover. Since these roles are all projections of the self, there is no need for someone else to actually sit there. In this context, the patient writes his "script," a dialogue between himself and the other person. He will reverse roles, actually changing chairs when he does this. It is important to note that the script the patient writes always takes place, as indicated in the "here and now" of Gestalt. There is no recreation of past encounters or preparations for future ones, as usually occurs in psychodrama.

In "dream work" in psychodrama, the protagonist will choose auxiliary egos to play other people, or images in his dream; while in Gestalt therapy, the patient again will play all the parts himself. The dream is entirely his creation and every art is a projection of himself. He tells the dream in the present and becomes every part, be it person or object. He writes a script in which the different parts have encounters with each other. Hopefully, the encounter will lead to conflict, then to mutual learning, understanding and appreciation of their differences, and finally to integration of the opposing forces. (It is, of course, also a recognized concept in psychodrama that the "other roles" played by auxiliary egos are essentially "extensions" of the protagonist's thoughts.)

Both psychodrama and Gestalt therapy have at least one common aim: self-actualization in a society in which most people dedicate their lives to actualizing a concept of what they should be like if they conform as robots. A crucial difference, however, as manifested by their different techniques, is Gestalt therapy's insistence that everything outside of ourselves is a projection and that growth lies in taking responsibility for those projections and owning up to them, so to speak. In psychodrama not everything is a self-projection: there are some consensual group realities, and some emphasis is given to the recognition of group norms and of the emotions of others in the group. In this regard, it is my contention that the Gestalt approach could benefit greatly by the application of the basic psychodramatic principles of involving *the group* more directly into the session. In psychodrama we often use the empty chair to represent a relevant other; however, there are times when the physical, verbal, and emotional amplification of the other by an actual other person in the form of an auxiliary ego will enormously enlarge the therapeutic benefit. For example, psychodramatic role reversal with an *actual* other person gives the protagonist a chance to (a) clarify how the significant other acts in real life for the director, group, auxiliary egos, and himself; (b) gives him an idea how it feels to be the significant other in the situation; and (c) gives him a chance to view himself from another prospective, through the significant others' eyes.

In many respects, we often encounter ourselves internally only at the level of our monodramas. Projecting our emotions onto an empty chair is of some value; however, the fiber and vibration of another person in psychodramatic auxiliary ego form enhances the intensity and scope of the exploration.

In Gestalt therapy, some of the sense of closeness and involvement is lost, since the "audience" remains an audience and is not involved in the acting-out process of the session. The group in Gestalt can only "identify" as observers and not fully as participants. In psychodrama people in the group experience a greater sense of involvement by playing auxiliary egos and doubles. Another aspect of the Gestalt situation is that it ties up the subject in every aspect of a session without a chance to observe others playing his role as an auxiliary ego would in psychodrama. The subject in Gestalt thus has no time to observe since he is always busy acting out all the various parts.

In both Gestalt therapy and Psychodrama, close attention is paid to body language; however, in psychodrama the use of an auxiliary ego in role reversal provides the subject with an opportunity to see his body-postures. We often have the auxiliary ego exaggerate movements so that the protagonist can better see how he looks in a situation. In psychodrama the director or aware double or auxiliary ego will use the body language observed to integrate the feeling projected into a session. For example, a double, observing that the protagonist's fists are clenched tightly, may speak for the subject in a tight, angry voice, to make the subject aware that those feelings are there but suppressed; the director, in sensing pent-up anger revealed by the protagonist's body tension, may have the subject act out the anger with a bottaca; and the auxiliary ego can mention the observed body language in the course of the session, such as, "You say that you forgive me but I see you keep hitting the chair and shaking your head at me."

In summary, the Gestalt approach could be considerably strengthened by involving the group more in the session through such psychodramatic techniques and elements as the auxiliary ego, the double, and the role reversal. In general, the production of a person's life script in a fuller, more dramatic fashion by using more psychodramatic techniques would help improve the theory and method of Gestalt therapy.

PRIMAL THERAPY *

The system and treatment of primal therapy, as developed by Dr. Arthur Janov, rests on the basic assumption that neurotic behavior is produced by "Primal Pain." He describes primal pain, in part, as "tension frozen in the body" that originates when the organisms (generally the infant's) psycho-physical needs are not met. For example, according to Janov, an unresolved primal condition can form in a child when it is not physically held enough, touched enough, or nursed according to its needs rather than on an external schedule. In brief, primal pain develops when the child's needs are not satisfied.

Janov postulates that the primal problem builds slowly as the child relinquishes his real needs and wants to the pressure of the external world, ultimately denying to himself that he has these needs. As a simplistic example, a child wants to be loved. It does

* For a comprehensive discussion of this modality see Arthur Janov, *The Primal Scream* (New York: G. P. Putnam's Sons, 1970).

not receive the love and attention it desires. Eventually, the child stops asking and blockades the pain of the need with a neurotic overlay that manifests itself in later life. A case example would be an actor for whom the most tumultous applause is insufficient because a basic approval desired was not received when he wanted it most as a child.

The therapeutic process of feeling primal pain, making the connect (between the pain and neurotic behavior), and exorcising the pain takes a few years of "primaling." By "primaling," the patient feels his pain and as a consequence "screams or cries" on a deep emotional level. To help a patient feel his pain, various devices are used that could be characterized as psychodramatic props. For example, baby bottles, six foot cribs and even machines designed to simulate birth experiences are used to help a patient confront his pain. Bags are punched and a whole range of primal physical activity is encouraged to facilitate a patient's feeling.

In primal therapy, as in psychodrama, patients are directed to *talk* to their parents rather than *about them;* and the primal therapist, like the psychodramatic director, attempts to facilitate real and deep feeling. In psychodramatic sessions, the goal of achieving a new and successful response to an old situation often materializes as a highly cathartic expression of feeling by the protagonist toward a significant other in his life. Although psychodrama does not limit the "successful response" to catharsis, there are many psychodramatic techniques that would be especially useful during the initial stages of primal therapy, when the primary objective is to break down the patient's defenses in order to reach deeper levels of feeling. A patient's role reversal with each of his parents, for example, could give the primal therapist a better picture of the patient's view of his parents and set the stage for deeper emotional explorations. The introduction of psychodrama can, in these ways, be a vital instrument for warming-up patients to their primal condition.

In this regard, Michael Solomon, who is a psychodramatist with extensive experience in primal therapy, stated in one of his lectures: "The flexibility of psychodrama is such that it can be structured to resemble a fairly traditional primal session and to even produce the kind of highly expressive catharsis often referred to as 'a primal.' This session would resemble an 'empty chair' Gestalt encounter except that even the chair would be missing. Instead the patient, alone with the psychodrama director, would describe a scene with the appropriate characters in it. As the description began to conjure anxiety or other feelings in the protagonist, the director would help the patient feel his past pain by encouraging him to speak directly to his internalized auxiliaries and then to watch and listen carefully to the imagined projected response. Other devices such as deep breathing, sinking into one's body or into a particularly tense area of the body, could also be employed by the director to achieve ever deeper expressions of feeling and releases of tension."

It is, of course, a historical fact that before Janov "discovered" the primal, the experience and the utilization of it for the treatment of neurosis were known to Freud and a host of other therapists. Moreno, in many areas of his discussion of psychodrama, has referred to the primal experience, but he used different terminology than Janov. My clarification of this historical fact is not in any way intended to undercut Janov's contribution in focusing the phenomenon of the primal and its treatment.

In hundreds of psychodrama sessions I have directed, protagonists have expressed their primal pain, made the connect, clarified their emotions, and in some measure resolved their problems. In this regard, I would assert that psychodrama is more potent for the protagonist because he is encouraged to react to the basic human source of his primal pain (mother, father, etc.) in the form of an auxiliary ego. Moreover, the situation that is constructed in psychodrama is closer than any other modality in delineating the original circumstances that produced the neurosis. The added dimension of the represented person (in an auxiliary ego form) in the psychodramatic situation provides a most fertile environment for achieving the primal response. The system developed and focused by Janov could effectively benefit from the incorporation of a range of psychodramatic concepts, especially the valuable use of the group, and techniques (especially role reversal, the double, and soliloquy) into the primal therapy approach.

TRANSACTIONAL ANALYSIS *

Psychiatrist Eric Berne was the originator of Transactional Analysis. He developed the treatment strategy of Transactional Analysis based on the assumption that all people bring to human interaction ("the transaction") three ego states:

1. PARENT: an ego state that resembles the parental figures who tell us how to do things and what we should and should not do. The parent ego state is the part of us that is judgmental and critical, Victorian, prejudiced, often quite bossy and opinionated. Parent' love is totally conditional: "I will love you if you do what I say." In the parent is stored prejudiced, antiquated, irrelevant beliefs that many people have never questioned. In brief, according to Transactional Analysis, everyone carries a "parent" around inside him.
2. ADULT: an ego state that is autonomously directed toward objective appraisal of reality, one that examines and evaluates. The adult state bases decisions on facts and is capable of objective data processing. In brief, the adult ego state is a computer that has the ability to be rational, to reason and calculate, to observe what is happening, and to take inner responsibility for one's actions.
3. CHILD: an active ego state that was fixated in childhood. It reflects the "I want to" feelings and emotions developed in childhood. The child ego state is the seat of all-powerful emotions—fear, anger, sadness, joy, elation, and playfulness. The child state is very aware of feelings and senses. Raw intuition is at a heightened state. Berne asserts that as the child develops, "this awareness of his senses is slowly trained out of him." His spontaneous "child" learns that in order to please those around him he must mask his natural feelings.

* The process of Transactional Analysis is comprehensively discussed in: Eric Berne, *Transactional Analysis in Psychotherapy* (New York: Grove Press, Inc., 1961) and Thomas Harris, *I'm O.K., You're O.K.* (New York: Harper & Row, 1969). I am grateful to Lenore Batiste, a student of both psychodrama and transactional analysis for her contribution to this section.

(This parallels Janov's theory of the development of primal pain and the psychodrama concept of developing robot behavior patterns.) Mother says, "Don't you talk to me that way. Stop carrying on and laughing so loud"; Father says, "You stop that crying this instant"; and the adapted child emerges. He must either rebel or comply; he does not have permission to feel freely for fear that he will no longer be loved and cared for. This repressed, hurt "child" is often carried around in the adult body.

The treatment in Transactional Analysis consists, in part, of effort to get PARENT, ADULT, and CHILD to work together and to allow ADULT to solve problems. The purpose of the adult is to separate itself from the other two ego states. One of the objects of Transactional Analysis is to enable people to use their appropriate ego state at any given moment in an apparent situation. The adult, for example, is activated when a person chooses to move from pain to joy, hate to love, or envy to admiration. The natural child acknowledges the feeling, says it's okay to have it, and then utilizes the adult to select the feeling that is appropriate for well-being. Transactional Analysis essentially attempts to free the "adult" to become effective in selecting a choice of action rather than to be imprisoned by archaic ideas and beliefs that have caused pain and confusion. According to Berne, to act in the most effective way you need "a decontaminated adult," i.e., an adult that is separate and independent of the other two ego states. In Transactional Analysis, people are educated to train their adult to give them information for appropriate action.

In Transactional Analysis, an important assertion is that "transactions" with people become much more effective if they are aware of which ego state they are operating in and which state is being activated within their self. If two people are in similar ego states, conversation can continue. In the Transactional Analysis lexicon, these similar ego states are called "parallel transactions" and they are complementary.

Everyone has a myriad of complex costumes (ego states) and they are activated at will. "Let's go to the beach and go swimming." "Yes, that would be fun," is a child-to-child parallel transaction. "How much did that dress cost?" "Thirty dollars," would be an adult-to-adult parallel transaction. Crossed transactions are carried out when people are operating from different ego states. These transactions will stop communication and can result in bad feelings. "How much did that dress cost?" may be a question asked by a husband of his wife to gain information, but if she views it as a critical parent question to her child, she may respond defensively with, "Did I ask you how much your tools cost?" This kind of communication, if continued, can erode a relationship that could otherwise be fulfilling if people were aware of their ego states and were operating on a parallel emotional level.

In Transactional Analysis terms, a *stroke* is a fundamental unit of social action. *An exchange of strokes is a transaction.* An objective of Transactional Analysis therapists is to teach people how to satisfy what is referred to as "stroke hunger" in positive ways. Strokes can be physical, visual, verbally empathetic, or praising. One can be stroked merely for "being," which is a deep and meaningful stroke, or for doing, which becomes conditional and not quite as penetrating. Transactional therapists believe that most of a person's basic motivation and action is to satisfy the hunger for strokes. When "the child" is not getting strokes, he becomes unhappy and frightened. People become addicted to certain ways of obtaining strokes. If they were stroked as children for acting helpless, hopeless, and depressed, they may resort to these tactics as adults. This could be called a "racket" and is used to manipulate other people. Eric Berne has popularized many of the games people play in order to receive strokes in his book *Games People Play*.

When interacting with others, transactions take the form of (1) rituals, (2) pastimes, (3) games, (4) intimacy, and (5) activity. Each person in interaction with others seeks as many satisfactions as possible from his transactions with others. The most prevalent social contacts are games and intimacy. Many games, in addition to attempting to acquire strokes, are ways of avoiding intimacy. In Transactional Analysis, the focus is on finding out which ego state (PARENT, ADULT, or CHILD) implements the stimulus and which provokes the response.

To attain autonomy, the individual must become game-free. He must overcome the programming of the past. The Transactional Analysis group is considered effective in analyzing transactions.

Transactional Analysis has been developed further by Dr. Thomas Harris in his book *I'm O.K. You're O.K.* Dr. Harris constructs four life positions based on his determination of the fundamental facets of Berne's ego state personalities: the child, the parent, and the adult. The individual, according to Harris, can view the parties in an interaction in four ways, and it is this recognition that tempers his response. The four ways of recognition are; (1) I'm not o.k., you're o.k.; (2) I'm o.k., you're not o.k.; (3) I'm not o.k., you're not o.k.; and (4) you're o.k., I'm o.k. The ideal method of association, of course, is I'm o.k., you're o.k., since the other combinations reflect themselves in dysfunctional interaction.

In the normal growth process, according to Harris, it is reasonable for the normal child to decide on I'm not o.k., you're o.k. This early position is fine; it indicates that there has been love, affection, and approval in the child's life but also indicates that he is at the mercy of others, basically his parents. To hold onto this position into adulthood is, of course, self-destructive. The second positions of I'm o.k., you're not o.k. is arrived at by the brutalized child who did not get enough love and approval. This would be the position that Al Capone or Adolf Hitler might have arrived at. This type of person can set up his own yes-men and get good strokes and approval, although in reality he is aware that the strokes are not genuine responses but motivated by fear. This ego position is very difficult to treat.

The third position, I'm not o.k., you're not o.k. is arrived at when the adult stops developing. In order for the adult to develop further, it is imperative that positive strokes are brought forward to encourage the adult. In Dr. Harris's Transactional Analysis terms, a person has arrived for the most part at the fourth position: "I'm o.k., you're o.k." This is a position in life where a person does not feel he is inferior, nor does he go through life viewing others as inferior to him. In brief, "I'm o.k., you're o.k." means that a person is secure enough to accept himself and others as they are, therefore producing a mutually beneficial relationship.

A later development of Transactional Analysis is encompassed in Claude Steiner's book *Scripts People Live By.* Dr. Steiner enlarges the "life script" concept Dr. Berne originated. As an example, he refers to the "witch mother" who infuses her child with a negative "self-fulfilling prophecy" fear. "You wait and see. You'll grow old just like me and you'll be poor, unhappy, and lonely, too." The child, Dr. Steiner asserts, often fulfills in life the negative script inculcated in this type of mother. His analysis of a variety of life scripts tends to enlarge the scope and meaning of Transactional Analysis.

Obviously, the foregoing is a rather brief and simplistic appraisal of the more highly developed Transactional Analysis system of therapy. Despite my perfunctory description, it is apparent that Transactional Analysis is a system of valid analysis of the games many people play to obfuscate their deeper emotions. Like psychoanalysis, the analytic system of Transactional Analysis has the merit of aiding both the professional and the patient to more closely examine their underlying motivations and to free themselves from neurotic behavior.

Psychodrama has been used as a helpful adjunct in Transactional Analysis both individually and in groups. The therapist suggests that the patient attempt an ongoing dialogue between his Parent, Child, and Adult. Three chairs are set up for this purpose, with the patient moving freely from one ego state to the other. After the Child and the Parent have interacted, the Adult is then activated to observe, evaluate, and select a plan of action. It has been observed that this inner dialogue is operating in each individual without his awareness much of the time. Therapists often advise their patients to use a tape recorder to verbally act out conversations between the three ego states. This technique is especially helpful to patients who may be too shy or repressed to adequately express their feelings in the therapist's office.

On one occasion, a sign was tacked up on the door outside a Transactional Analysis group therapy session that read "No one over seven years old allowed inside." People who had difficulty expressing negative or positive feelings toward each other found it much easier to do so by roleplaying their seven-year-old child ego state. This role-playing device produced many emotions and resulted in raucous laughter and tears over the span of the three-hour session.

In some groups, people who have difficulty confronting a critical Parent figure or haven't the inner resources to activate their own adult can respond psychodramatically to each other. The therapist may be seen as a nurturing Parent surrounded by a group of free children, and much of the repressed spontaneous Child is able to emerge in this psychodramatically induced environment.

So-called permission workshops have arisen in the Transactional Analysis community. In this context, the therapist gives everyone permission to act freely as spontaneous children. Children's games are played, direct eye contact between people is encouraged, and trustworthy parents are set up to escort blindfolded children around the environment. Reenacting birth or enacting death are often found to be insight-provoking experiences. In Transactional Analysis, another psychodramatic technique called psycho-sculpture is utilized. In this process, a patient creates a sculptural sociogram of his family or social group, physically lacing members where he sees them emotionally. Once he observes where he has placed them, he can then move them around to where he would like them to be. In addition to being entertaining, this process allows people to gain more insight into their family and social relationships.

There appear to be several additional ways in which the Transactional Analysis process can be further enhanced by the use of psychodrama. Psychodrama can help articulate the three ego states of parent, child, and adult by having a protagonist enact a specific scene in his life when the ego-states are explicated by actual life roles, or when one of the states was apparently dominant in interaction with another. The sessions should use others as auxiliary egos. I would recommend that Transactional Analysis use psychodrama in the client's early therapeutic sessions. This would provide the Transactional Analysis analyst and the client with a more direct appraisal of each ego state as it relates to the client's life. An added benefit in using psychodrama is that an ego state can be understood in the context of the more specific socialization situations that nurture its development. For example, in a session I directed with a young lady, whose "child" was deprived when she was young, she acted out a scene in which she sought love from her parents. In the session, they explicitly and dramatically denied her need. She exploded in tears. She determinedly let this set of experiences dominate her life by an "I'm not o.k., you're o.k." perspective. We then had her act out a scene with her husband that approximated an I'm o.k., you're o.k. situation. In the post-discussion, we discussed the relationships between the two scenes and in later sessions attempted to reinforce more of her adult ego state scenarios.

In a like manner, I would suggest that a Transactional Analysis therapist, in early sessions, have clients psychodramatically act out a scene depicting each position of: (1) I'm not o.k., you're o.k.; (2) I'm not o.k., you're not o.k.; (3) I'm o.k., you're not o.k.; and finally (4) I'm o.k., you're o.k. As the therapy progresses, the client will increasingly enact scenes from the fourth position. This might be done to solidify and reinforce behavior in this posture.

In brief, the central way psychodrama can be a useful adjunct to Transactional Analysis is to make more explicit *in action* those aspects of behavior that are interpreted and analyzed *verbally* in Transactional Analysis. Through this live enactment aspect, psychodrama can help enlarge the meaning and success of the Transactional Analysis system.

REALITY THERAPY *

Reality Therapy, as developed by Dr. William Glasser, is based on the assumption that people must confront their reality, responsibility, and their concepts of right and wrong in order to be emotionally healthy. In this context, problems are a manifestation of a person's inability to fulfill his needs in the present. The past is, in Reality Therapy terms, "historical garbage." In brief, irrational or inadequate behavior is viewed as an effort to cope with and solve the discomfort and misery brought about by failure to fulfill one's needs in relationship to one's personal reality in the present.

According to Glasser, a common characteristic of people in trouble is to deny the reality of the world around them. Whether that denial is partial or total, it is common to all patients. The variations of this denial as described by Glasser include: breaking the law, paranoid claims of being plotted against; fear of close quarters, airplanes, height, elevators; fear of existent situations; excessive drinking; and the use of drugs. Glasser states this premise about clients, "No matter what behavior they choose, all patients have a common characteristic: *They all deny the reality of the world around them.* . . . Whether it is a partial denial or the total blotting out of all reality of the chronic backward patient in the state hospital, the denial of some or all of reality is common to all patients. Therapy will be successful when they are able to give up denying the world and recognize that reality not only exists but that they must fulfill their needs within its framework."

Reality Therapy attempts to lead the client toward successfully coping within the framework of the real world of norms and to fulfill his needs so that there is no further inclination for denial of reality's existence. In order to achieve this goal, according to Glasser, two basic needs must be recognized: "to be loved and to feel worthwhile." Is this regard, he asserts that everyone must

---

* For a comprehensive presentation and analysis of Reality Therapy see William Glasser's book *Reality Therapy* (New York: Harper Colophon Books, 1965).

be involved with other people to fulfill their needs. To be helped in Reality Therapy, the patient must achieve involvement, first with the therapist and then with others.

According to Dr. Glasser, the ability of the therapist to get involved is the major skill of doing Reality Therapy. To understand how this involvement occurs, certain qualities are necessary to the therapist. He must be "responsible, tough, interested, human, and sensitive." He must be willing to discuss some of his own struggles so that the patient can see that acting responsibly is possible though sometimes difficult. He must have the strength to become involved, to have his values tested by the patient, and to withstand intense criticism by the patient. He must always be strong, never expedient. To some extent, he must be affected by the patient and his problems and even suffer with him (a form of doubling). In this area of full involvement, the role of the Reality Therapy therapist and the psychodramatist are parallel, since in psychodrama all members of the group as well as the director are expected to become emotionally involved with the psychodramatic protagonist.

In summary, Glasser's Reality Therapy stresses six basic points:

1. The concept of mental illness is not accepted; therefore, the patient cannot become involved with Reality Therapy as a mentally ill person who has no responsibility for his behavior.
2. Patients relate to therapists as themselves, not as transference figures. The Reality Therapy therapist attempts to exclude the possibility of transference and insists on a direct relationship with the client.
3. The Reality Therapy therapist works in the present and toward the future with no involvement in the patient's history. Since it cannot be changed, the Reality Therapy therapist does not accept the fact that a patient is limited by his past.
4. The Reality Therapy therapist disregards unconscious conflicts or reasons for them. Glasser takes the position that a patient cannot become involved with the therapist by excusing his behavior on the basis of unconscious motivations.
5. Emphasis is placed on the morality of behavior. The issue of right and wrong is faced by both therapist and client.
6. Patients are directly taught better ways to fulfill their needs.

The Reality Therapist defines his role as a teacher and gives specific advice on moral issues and states specific positive ways for dealing with problems.

Glasser considers the acting-out of experiences and feelings as damaging to the therapy; he feels that such enactment would tend to reinforce a patient's "irresponsible" behavior and attitudes.

In psychodrama, of course, acting-out is central to the therapy and the group is more fundamental to a session. In psychodrama the therapeutic role is not as totally focused on the director as in Reality Therapy; the therapeutic responsibility is spread throughout the therapeutic group. Each member in the session, including the therapist, contributes to the definition and judgment of what is reality. Additionally, the emotional material presented is not restricted to the present. The acting-out of past, present, and future is considered crucial to the therapeutic process in psychodrama.

Psychodrama, therefore, is able to treat problematic experiences in a multi-dimensional rather than uni-dimensional fashion. The "surplus reality" setting that the psychodramatic group can create allows the members of the group to test all the nuances not only of their present attitudes and behavior but also of the potential effects of different possible approaches to their social relationships. In a certain sense, the group in a psychodramatic situation provides a greater reality than in Reality Therapy. The psychodramatic setting is advantageous in that it formulates the formation of a many-channeled social network that more closely approximates the number and types of mutual relationships characteristic of a person's real social atom. Unlike Reality Therapy, the group has a primary validity and group members are encouraged to participate in each other's treatment. In psychodrama the group impact is a reality that cannot be theoretically ignored because it is empirically a vital force in the procedure.

Another contrast between psychodrama and Reality Therapy is related to the goals inherent in the methods. The Reality Therapist defines "reality and realistic behavior" and adjustment to the norms of society as a desirable goal. Psychodrama, however, uses a dynamic definition of reality that allows for the personal interpretation of a situation to affect how each person will respond. Protagonists are encouraged *not* to simply follow established normative patterns but to create for themselves the response that will be most effective in a situation. In reverse, it appears that the Reality Therapy approach tends to reinforce culturally conserved responses, justifying this reinforcement as appropriate to an unchanging social reality. Giving "future shock" some credence, culture and society are obviously not static and the speed of social change has been accelerating. It is not more routinization that a person needs but an enhancement of his spontaneity and creativity to act so that he relates more effectively to the novel situations that dynamic contemporary life repeatedly generates.

Reality Therapy could benefit from a variety of role-playing techniques that would inject greater reality into the process. For example, in its own context, when a client is talking about his reality, the therapist could double for him, thus adding *his* perspective to the client's reality. It would also seem useful as an adjunct to Reality Therapy in group settings to have various members of the group help a person discussing his reality by playing the roles of significant others. This might sharpen the client's concept of reality. Although the Reality Therapy client's concept of the past "as garbage" might be maintained, it would seem useful to explore some of these situations through role-playing for the purpose of correcting past errors. It would also seem most useful to have a client reverse roles with his therapist, if only for the therapist to validate in what ways the client has learned his reality lessons.

A further technique that could be utilized by the Reality Therapist would be the use of the psychodramatic role test. The therapist and the client could delineate several areas of significant relearning, and then the client could be role-tested for his future performance in these areas in order to evaluate the meaning of his new-found reality. For example, a former drug addict client concludes that his drug-taking has been clearly self-destructive. It would be useful as a psychodramatic reality test to have an auxiliary ego in a role-playing situation offer him some drugs. The role test would revolve around the effectiveness of his response. The positive effect of the treatment could thus be corroborated. Such testing is required, because in Reality Therapy, contrary to its emphasis, there is no true testing of reality; the therapist has only the verbal testimony of the client that he has changed. The introduction of psychodrama offers a hypothetical "surplus reality" setting in which the patient can safely explore all possibilities before attempting a different pattern of behavior in the real world. The adjunctive use of psychodrama in Reality Therapy provides an opportunity to more closely examine the client's perceptions of reality and to role test any therapeutic advancement that the client appears to have accomplished. Also a broader use of the group would serve as an *in situ* test of therapeutic progress of the client.

Another more recent development of Glasser's concept of Reality Therapy is developed in his book *Schools Without Failure*. Glasser notes that most schools in the central areas of cities process children for failure because their educational programs are "irrelevant and do not provide methods for effectively involving children in the educational process." Children react to this failure with withdrawal and often delinquent behavior. Glasser's central thesis is that "if a child, no matter what his background can succeed in school, he has an excellent chance for success in life." He asserts that teachers should become in effect, Reality Therapists—they should "offer friendship understanding and get involved with helping children overcome their emotional problems." To accomplish this, he recommends that every subject taught should be related to something the child acts out in his day-to-day life inside and outside of school.

In this regard, psychodrama related to both curriculum and personal problems is a method that can involve children more effectively than most discussion techniques. Psychodrama relevantly applied in the classroom situation can counterattack the conditions producing emotional problems that emerge later in life.

Psychodrama in the Classroom

Psychodrama has been utilized at every level of the educational system, from kindergarten to the post-graduate seminar. The sessions have been related not only to subject matter but to current social events, "character development," and emotional problems.

Not everyone is an advocate of psychodrama in the classroom, and the practice is of sufficient social political importance to agitate former Vice President Spiro T. Agnew. In a speech in 1971 delivered to the Illinois Agricultural Association, he commented:

> Perhaps you have heard of the so-called "psycho-dramas" that children of all ages are forced to act out in the classroom. Listen to this account that I read recently in a newspaper: ". . . teachers frequently ask them [the pupils] to act out such things as obtaining an abortion, interracial dating, smoking marijuana—and how their parents would react. Parents find even more objectionable "psychodramas" in which children act out actual incidents from the home, something which parents consider a clear invasion of their privacy. There have also been "talk-ins" where two or three children will go to the school counselor and answer highly personal questions, such as: "What does your father wear when he shaves?" or "Do you love your parents?" One child was assigned an essay on the subject, "Why do I hate my mother more than my father?"
>
> Character that was once molded in the home is now more often the product of the classroom, and there are some who would like to take it a step further and indoctrinate or condition all preschool age children from infants on up to kindergarten age. They admire the Soviet system in which the State takes over this function from the parent.

The debate over teachers dealing with a child's emotional state in class—beyond the curriculum—is still a controversial issue in many school systems. Despite this, the application of role-playing that relates to emotional problems has become an established practice in the classroom. Psychodrama is utilized in the classroom for both the child's emotional growth and for curriculum purposes on subject matter. In connection with transmitting information, many teachers use a wide array of role-playing techniques.

Many teachers have role-playing sessions in which children (after being informed on a subject) psychodramatically assume the role of the inanimate or animate object they are studying. To understand the subject or role on a deeper level, a child may become a tree or an animal, or assume the role of police-officer, lawyer, doctor, mayor, president.

In the same vein, role-playing has been effectively employed in teaching such subjects as literature and history. In literature, when reading a story, it is useful to act out the central figures in the story so that the student can develop a deeper emotional understanding of the character and, to a degree, himself. For example, young children in the early grades might become Snow White or each of the seven dwarfs and discuss the reason why they are Dopey, Grumpy, Sleepy, Sneezy, Happy, Doc, or Bashful. The simple procedure of asking a student why he would like to play a particular character can also produce insights into his personality. Each child in the process of playing his character should soliloquize his personal feelings as the character. Other literary works that have broad implications for role-playing and character development are Lewis Caroll's Alice in Wonderland and the Wizard of Oz. In sessions I have run with teenagers, the session invariably veers off into a discussion of psychedelic drugs. Was Alice or Judy Garland's Dorothy high on acid?

On a deeper level, at the junior high and high school level, such classics as *Moby Dick, Hamlet, Macbeth, Catcher In the Rye, The Sun Also Rises,* or *The Grapes of Wrath* provide springboards for insightful psychodramatic performance. I would suggest that the literature and the characters be acted out in a free style that facilitates the student's development of spontaneity and gives him a broad range for interpretation. For example, consider the possibilities of the "To be or not to be" scene from *Hamlet*. In a session I ran with high school age students, it kicked off an exciting and useful examination of the social implications of suicide.

History can be made exciting and interesting through role-playing that goes beyond the surface into emotional issues. Portraits of significant periods and episodes in history tend to personally and emotionally stimulate student involvement. For example, in examining patriotic emotions, it might be useful in lieu of saluting the flag to have a different child, each day, role-play "the flag" and talk about such issues as how he came into existence and what he stands for. Dialogue with the "student-flag" should, of course, be encouraged. This type of psychodramatic interaction would breathe some life into a role ritual that no longer has much meaning for most children.

In a deeper historical context, have a student play George Washington, Abraham Lincoln, Franklin D. Roosevelt, John F. Kennedy, or Richard Nixon and present each former president's speeches. Have students (black and white) play blacks of that era and militants of today as the audience to the speech. Properly done, this type of session will veer into a psychodrama on the role of a president or contemporary race relations between students and will reveal some of the emotions young people have about these issues.

On a more direct emotional level, psychodrama sessions in the classroom can encompass such subjects as dating, meeting new people, envying others, not having lots of clothes (or the right clothes), getting low grades, being embarrassed to speak in front of the class, getting high grades on tests, making a mistake in front of the class, being complimented, having money stolen, cheating on tests, gossiping, running for school office, taking drugs, sexual promiscuity, vandalism, losing in a contest, being absent from school frequently, losing one's possessions, forgetting things, not completing assignments, and fair and unfair discipline by the teachers.

The psychodrama sessions can utilize the following order of

action: (1) first have students select and discuss a problem as a warm-up; (2) assign roles according to the problem situation; (3) enact a specific situation involving the tensions and conflict; (4) analyze patterns of conflict that appear in the role-playing; and (5) replay for better relationships and improved role performance.

One teacher's report on her role-playing in the classroom reveals the broad range of subjects covered and the practice involved.

> With the younger pre-school children my "games" are painless "let's pretend" although I do like to ask the children the whys of the profession they choose and also to try to have the significant others present (i.e., doctors and nurses, football players and spectators or coaches, teachers, and, of course, students). In all these role-playing experiences I feel the children are being creative, however, with the primary grade children I go one step further. Instead of just "playing" roles I have them reverse roles. One that seems to be the favorite is that boys are girls and girls are boys, or children from different ethnic or racial groups reverse roles. When the children are finished at playing each other I ask them to share what it *felt* like. I like to know if they would like to always be a boy (girls), black (white), parent (child), teacher (student), or if they were glad it was a game. Most indicate they like their real role.
>
> This technique can be very helpful in disciplinary action. If a child is really making a lot of disturbance or is hurting another child I use role reversal with the child and myself or let the two children do it. Of course this involves a short explanation of the theory and method, but I try to let them confront each other as soon as possible in role-playing after the fight. I have often thought that when I am having a particularly crabby day it would be good for me to let one of the children reverse roles with me, but my courage has not permitted this as yet. If by using these techniques I am able to encourage the humanness in my children, then the rewards are self-evident.

The potential of the use of psychodrama in schools among those children who are having learning and social problems is illustrated by a psychodrama experiment conducted in a New

York school with a class of eighteen so-called maladjusted boys, all of whom had average-to-above-average intelligence. Of the eighteen boys, ten were confirmed truants and most had been involved in petty theft or vandalism. All of the boys were aggressive and many were prone to acting-out violence. All of the boys were performing well below standard in school, were discouraged easily in school, and then either cut school, lost their temper, fought, or stole. All of the boys in the study tended to be disruptive and undisciplined in the classroom. Whenever they ran up against a situation they could not handle, they became antagonistic and quarrelsome, sulked, walked around the room, and generally interfered with other children who were working.

In applying psychodrama to their learning situations, it was not merely a matter of getting a selfish boy to play a generous role, or a cowardly child a heroic role, although this appeared to have value, but rather to present the children with situations in their daily lives which trouble them and to which they responded inadequately. It was recognized that positive change in these boys could not be achieved in just one session. As a consequence of many psychodrama sessions, there were improved social responses in the various situations these boys confronted daily in their home, family, and school life. In five weeks some remarkable changes were noted in the behavior of most of the boys. By the end of the school term, they showed better attitudes, developed improved relationships with classmates, had greater self-discipline, and markedly improved class attendance and work.

Using psychodrama with problem children in school is much more effective if the children's parents can be involved. As part of a delinquency prevention program I ran in New York in the mid-fifties, I introduced this approach with positive results. The project took place at P.S. 93 in Manhattan, a school located in an urban area beset by the many complex and extreme problems of contemporary society. We attempted to select out, for the project, the parents of the most difficult problem children in the school. The determination of who these students were was simply handled by having the principal and a panel of ten teachers list their "top twenty troublemakers." Interestingly, there was remarkable consensus in identifying these students. The principal then invited the parents of these problem children to "become part of a group exploring children's problems in school."

The group met one night a week for a six-month period. Most of the parents (fathers and mothers) attended regularly. We moved into such role-playing situations as disciplining children, good and bad teachers, and a range of personal family problems. A report was written at the end of the program that summarized the following therapeutic effects:

1. Parents felt free to "blast" the school, within the group. Some catharsis was observed as well as some understanding about the fact that they were in many cases projecting onto the school their own limitations as parents.
2. Parents seemed to benefit from the knowledge that other parents had problems similar to theirs.
3. Parents found they could help each other to understand and resolve conflict situations by acting-out and discussing their experiences in the group. They agreed that more dimensions of a problem were brought to light in the role-playing than in their discussions. Moreover, the discussion parts of the session were more dynamic after role-playing.
4. Many recommendations and suggestions about methods and techniques for positively dealing with their children emerged in the group as a result of the role-playing; and the group gave its support to those parents who wanted to try them out.
5. The group established parent behavior norms. Permissive and punitive disciplinary approaches were acted out with the extremes tending to give way to more moderate approaches.

I have often used psychodrama in my college classroom. For example, in my criminology courses, after exploring a concept such as the "criminal psychopath," I would have a student come forward and play the role. The class would ask the student-psychopath a variety of interesting and self-revealing questions.

In analyzing the role of police in the community, I have students role-play police officers in various activities (e.g. giving a traffic ticket, breaking up a family fight, arresting a murderer, etc.). In one session I brought in members of the Gay Student Union on campus to confront a real police officer playing the role of the police chief opposed to the hiring of homosexuals for the police department. The session was highly emotional and revealed the variety of community prejudices and postures on the subject.

In exploring crime causation, in the classroom, I often get a student-protagonist who is courageous enough to admit to a delinquent act in his past. In one session I directed, at the height of an act of teenage burglary, I had the student-thief-protagonist freeze in the moment of the role and soliloquize his motivations. I then had other volunteer students double with his soliloquy. It is interesting to note that almost a third of the students in classes where I have presented this type of psychodrama come forward one by one and soliloquize a parallel act and their motivations. The process seems to make the subject more interesting, but more importantly, it provides an opportunity for a student to personally and emotionally identify with the subject.

During the political crisis of the past decade, in my sociology classes at California State University, Northridge, we carried out psychodramas on such issues as Watergate, Agnew's resignation, the 1968 Chicago police riots, the pardoning of Richard Nixon, and the crisis of New York City. Some of the most emotional and productive psychodramas revolved around Vietnam War veterans who enacted their emotions about their participation in the war. Many had residual feelings of great guilt about what they did during the war—and emotional aftershocks about having been exploited by their participation in the war.

One student, a woman in her forties, vividly described in a paper her first classroom psychodrama, which was provoked by issues connected to the war. Her psychodrama occurred in the context of a period of high emotional tension on campus, the day after the Kent State student murders by the national guard in Ohio. She was apathetic to the news she received about the event through usual channels, but the psychodrama process had a profound impact on her in giving the incident emotional meaning, psychodramatically changing her point of view and provoking direct social action:

My introduction to psychodrama came about in a rather unusual way. It happened during the period of the Kent State crisis. While taking a midterm exam in one of my classes a strike was raging through the halls. The ferocity of the student mob running in the halls had a frightening violence about it. I was terrified. I hated the violence on our campus. I arrived at my next class completely disoriented, frightened, angry, determined that no dissenter could take me from my seat in class. The professor had arranged for the class to be involved in a psychodrama that day. The director asked four students to lay on the floor and be the four Kent students who had been killed. Suddenly their death became very personal to me. I sat in my seat crying, feeling as though I was dying. I was asked to sit on the stage and tell the four dead students why I had reacted as I had and how I felt about them.

The drama progressed with auxiliary egos, Jerry Rubin, National Guardsmen, and myself. It was highly dramatic and you could feel the flow of heavy emotions throughout the classroom. Every person in that room was caught up in the drama that was being portrayed on the stage. We were bonded to each other, caught in the emotional forces that stripped us of isolated entity. For me, the climax came when, in the role of Jerry Rubin, I turned on the auxiliary ego *playing me* and called her a middle-class bitch who professed to love humanity but did nothing about it. When the class and the psychodrama ended I went back to my home raging with energy. I stalked in, confronted my poor unsuspecting husband, and told him that I didn't care what he thought or said but that I was getting *involved!* I became active in the strike at school doing whatever seemed appropriate to express my opinions. Apart from this involvement I joined an activist group that I had previously declined to join because I wished to avoid involvement. I became submerged in a group that attempted to cope with the problems that plagued our split generations. I delved into the drug problem, the abortion problem, problems of loneliness, lack of communication, and many others. As a result of that one psychodrama I felt more alive and became part of the mainstream of community life on campus and in the world.

As a professor of sociology over the past twenty-five years, I have taught a course on the subject of psychodrama almost every semester. The course always involves actual sessions with students. The discussion of sociological concepts is invariably enriched by a psychodrama session. For example, it seems arid to present a lecture on role theory without actually involving students in some scene in their life that related to communication, empathy, or the socialization process. In teaching all of these concepts, various psychodramatic techniques seem to be intrinsic vehicles to help the student understand basic concepts. In exploring role theory, for example, the Charles Horton Cooley concept of the "Looking Glass Self" or the G. H. Mead theory of empathy or "taking the role of the other" is actualized and explicated when a student psychodramatically reverses roles, doubles, or becomes an auxiliary ego.

One of my most exciting experiences with psychodrama in the classroom occurred during the height of the revolutionary student situation at California State University, Northridge, in 1968. Our campus was at times literally "exploding" with bombings, and a fire was set one night in the Administration Building. In protest for a larger enrollment of minority groups and a black studies program, there was at one point a takeover of the Administration Building that involved the forced captivity of about eight administrative university officers as hostages to obtain the student demands.

It was during the height of this series of episodes that I conceived an idea about utilizing psychodrama in an effort to diffuse the social bomb that had emerged on our campus and to help produce positive social change. As chairman of the Sociology Department, I was in a position to *quietly* set up a special "course in psychodrama." I selected the top fifteen or twenty most militant minority group and S.D.S. students on campus and personally invited them to participate in the course. I was successful in attracting about one third of these students plus around fifteen additional militant students to take the course. I further balanced out the class with another dozen students selected at random to provide a cross-section of position and opinion. Over the semester, at each class meeting, we had intense psychodramatic sessions that encompassed every facet of the campus conflict as well as a microcosm of many aspects of the macrocosmic civil rights movement in America.

The most dramatic session involved several black student leaders spewing out their deep rage against other members of the group who psychodramatically portrayed various authority figures, including the governor and President. The high point of the session occurred when the most militant black leader on campus reversed roles, became "the governor," and slowly, methodically, and brilliantly espoused "the governor's" apparent racist position. The session resulted in a most productive interchange of theoretical and philosophical ideas—beyond the former stale, rote rhetoric of militancy.

Other sessions explored the problems both minority students and professors were having with the influx of minority students ill-prepared in a variety of ways to do college-level work; the real and fantasized fears white students had about potential violence from militants; the deep insecurities felt by minority students that were hidden under their tough exterior; the militant extortion of high grades from professors by actual and implied threats of violence; and a range of usual student problems with higher education.

One unusual session was enacted by a militant black female student. She got into a standard session of premarital dating and mate selection. In one encounter with an auxiliary ego playing the role of her militant black boyfriend, she surprised herself and the group by finally, vehemently telling him: "Sucker, you're the last one in the world I'd ever want to settle down with and marry. You're a great dude at what you're trying to accomplish, but sometimes you scare me with how crazy you are. You're going to get your black ass killed by a pig one of these days. I want the father of any baby I have to have a solid job and some financial security." The student revealed that under her role of a "by any means necessary revolutionary exterior," she had a streak of typical, white, middle-class Americana.

In brief, the adjunct use of a range of psychodramatic concepts in education at all levels helps to resolve regular and complex educational problems, can serve as an aid to transmitting standard educational material, and can enliven the day-to-day procedures of the classroom so that it becomes a more attractive and enjoyable human situation.

There are many other institutional situations and treatment modalities utilizing psychodramatic techniques that have not been covered in this analysis. An innovative teacher or practitioner of individual or group psychotherapy can, however, creatively select some useful concepts or techniques from the foregoing discussion for utilization and adaptation to his or her specific work. Moving on from professional applications, in the ensuing discussion, I will explore the broader applications of psychodrama for non-professional use in the family, small impromptu groups, and as psychological theater for a mass audience.

CHAPTER
5

Psychodrama in Your Life: Impromptu Groups and Mass Theater

A studio is the abode of a unique enterprise. This is the Impromptu Theater, in which the acts have no lines to memorize and no rehearsals to undergo. In fact, everything is impromptu —the dramatists, the plays, the actors, the music, the dancing and even the "props."

Impromptu acting, according to Dr. Moreno, . . . is a preparation to meet the exigencies of life with calm and poise.

"Actual life," he says, "consists of endless sequences of unexpected and hence impromptu situations, and these are not chosen by the individual; they happen to him. In these situations the person either may follow a blind habit and obey the mechanism established in former experiences, or he may act spontaneously, radically modifying the mechanism, under the stimulus of the master key, his creative urge. . . ."

. . . Impromptu is an antidote for the machine age, a remedy for the robot. It aims to jerk men and women from the rut of a standardized existence, confronting them with unusual and unexpected situations which awaken their natural creative urge.

—*New York Sun,* August 8, 1930

EVERYONE is an actor. A select few recite lines written by someone else on a stage set. All people perform in everyday life. Most people's lines and postures are their own, culled forth spontaneously, essentially in standardized cultural situations.

There are three basic forms of human acting: *everyday life; theater;* and *psychodrama.* Most people (even professional actors) spend most of their time performing in *everyday life.* The second major arena of human performance is in *theater.* People spend a great deal of their time in this model of interaction, whether the performance is on stage or in a more passive role of a member of the audience. The audience is a vital element in any theatrical performance—and it is from this posture that most people participate in theater.

Psychodrama as a form of performance, when learned, is easier to enact since the actor is mainly asked to present his *real self*—even more than he does in everyday life. In daily life, the exigencies of a job, or other roles, often requires the masking and inhibition of certain emotions, whereas performance in psychodrama requires both the revelation of the external and the internal range of emotions.

Despite this factor of a more total self-presentation, psychodrama is a form of human behavior that occupies the least amount of time in most people's lifestyle. Yet, it has the potential for enriching the *existence* of people in at least equal measure to theater participation (actor or audience) and augmenting the satisfaction of everyday life. In this context, psychodrama is not only a therapeutic device or vehicle for solving human problems but also a form for interesting, satisfying, and significant human expression that can enrich and enlarge a person's existential condition. It provides the opportunity for a person to break out of the ordinary role-bound cultural models and experience new and different emotional states of being.

Sessions are usually most potent when they are directed by a trained psychodramatist; however, there are a variety of ways in which psychodrama can be useful and psychologically productive to relatively normal people (who are already born actors) in a variety of more natural and accessible group settings. In this regard, I would like to first summarize the possible ways for psychodrama to become part of your life. After delineating these possibilities, I will focus on those areas not yet fully discussed.

There are basically five general arenas for your participation in psychodrama:

1. In classic psychodrama sessions performed in a psycho-drama theater with a trained psychodramatist directing;
2. As you already have, in reading this book. In this regard, to some degree you have been (hopefully) able to personally immerse yourself in the scenarios of sessions presented here and have related these experiences to your own life with some beneficial impact;
3. The integration of psychodrama into situations in which another treatment modality is the central therapeutic approach. In this context, psychodrama is utilized as an adjunct to the dominant therapy by a therapist who is not necessarily accredited as a psychodramatist;
4. Informal, impromptu groups developed spontaneously in your family or community with the sessions directed by a designated member of the group;
5. Psychodrama sessions focusing on significant social issues transmitted to a mass audience in an auditorium, through television, in your home or on film in a theater.

So far the emphasis has been on the first three categories of participation as related to classical psychodrama. From here on I will focus on the latter possibilities with emphasis in the final two chapters on the broader theoretical implications and meaning of psychodrama as a theater of life.

Impromptu Group Psychodrama

A new direction in therapy is the support given by many professional therapists to self-help programs varyingly referred to as nonprofessional, leaderless, and informal therapy groups. The acceptance of the validity of these programs is related to the success and growth of such pioneer self-help efforts as Alcoholics Anonymous, Synanon, and other "nonprofessional" therapies. Many qualified professionals who have related to these groups as consultants and participants are enthusiastic about the positive results achieved in these therapeutic settings. This development dovetails with the apparent fact that the majority of people's personal problems and conflicts are discussed, analyzed, and often resolved by laymen in the normal settings of family, work, and community.

In brief, most people confronted with the normal problems of contemporary life do not discuss their difficulties with a psychotherapist. In fact, most problems that develop between family, friends, or at work can more often than not be resolved through discussion and counseling with the people related to each other in natural or self-help groups. In this context, I would suggest that psychodrama can be included as a valuable tool for enlarging and improving the informal counseling and discussions that already take place in such organic settings as the family, school, work, and the community. Psychodrama, therefore, infused into these natural group settings, can provide an interesting humanistic experience and can serve as a valuable vehicle for the analysis and resolution of the normal problems of everyday life outside of a formal therapeutic setting.

A psychodrama in the more informal impromptu setting requires a group of people who are in agreement to seriously utilize the psychodrama method for working on some of the problems and conflicts in their life. It is important to attempt to have one or more people in your group who have some knowledge of or training in human behavior concepts. It is also recommended that everyone in the group closely read this book on psychodrama so that they will be knowledgeable about the theory and method. All members should also agree that they will participate in the group for at least a series of five sessions. Some groups may flourish in the first session, but in most cases it takes several sessions for people to warm up to each other within the framework of the method.

In this discussion, I will not attempt to precisely define the exact way the group should proceed; however, certain general principles are applicable to all sessions. One caveat to observe is that all members of the group gathered together for a session for a defined period of time (two to four hours) should recognize that they are not engaged in a fun-and-games venture. There are many humorous and entertaining incidents that emerge in a session (as they do in life), but it should be made clear that the central purpose of the psychodrama is the group exploration of mutual dilemmas, problems, and conflicts.

A first step in an impromptu group psychodrama session is to briefly have all members of the group introduce themselves (even if they already know each other). In their introduction, they should try to state, as best they can, the problem area they would want to focus on if they became the protagonist in a session. This has the effect of warming people up to themselves in the here and now. The "director" and members of the group should then begin to further discuss aspects of their lives that they might want to explore. The session could center on husband-wife-lover conflicts, parent-child relationships, difficulties on the job, in-law problems, or emotions about larger social issues (living newspaper events). In this informal way, the group members should determine what human area they feel they want to focus on.

Larger social issues are less complex for a group than more basic interpersonal conflicts. For example, in exploring emotions about politics, a sense of hopelessness or helplessness in controlling one's destiny in a complex world, a member of the group could play the role of the president, governor, or some other public figure in the headlines; and the group could confront this significant image with their positive or negative feelings.

Another way to warm up the group for relevant action would be to take one of the scenarios from the preceding chapters, have members of the group *select* the roles they want to play, and then act out the life script. The process would tend to generate some emotional action and personalized post-discussion. This warm-up is useful in itself; however, it could lead to a more specific session with a member of the group.

On a more direct personal level, a member of the group might start the session with an enactment of an immediate conflict in his life. For example, "a common argument" that a couple repeatedly has, or some issue of child-rearing that members of the group feel is relevant. A pertinent scene that everyone can relate to is the enactment of the parental disciplining of a child, or a couple discussing their future together. In all cases, auxiliary egos should play the relevant other, and the designated director should, when he feels it is appropriate, provide doubles and have the protagonists reverse roles.

An innovative spontaneous group can have productive sessions by setting aside a regular time for meeting. The same group meeting on a regular basis will tend to grow more functional and creative with each session.

On a more spontaneous basis, people who have been participants in impromptu psychodrama groups can begin to have sessions in actual every day family situations, when it seems appropriate. For example, when (in our judgment) our son encounters a problem, my wife and I have a session with him on the spot. As an illustration of this, one day he came home from a fight at school complaining about a boy who was "always" picking on him. My wife directed and I played the "bully." After zeroing in on the situation, in which I as the "bully" beat him up, my wife had us reverse roles. When my son played the "bully," he was asked why he picked "on poor, innocent Mitch." As the "bully," he detailed the way Mitch provoked him to hit him. In the original story he told us, we heard very little about Mitch's role in the fight. The session helped him learn more about his role in the conflict and no doubt affected his future performance in such situations.

My wife, Donna, further enlarged Mitch's social insight into the fight by asking him several other questions, with him in the role of the "bully."

DONNA: Why are you always in trouble?
MITCH AS BULLY: I like to fight and beat kids up.
DONNA: But why?
MITCH AS BULLY: It's fun.
DONNA: Yes, but what's wrong with your life that makes you so angry?
MITCH AS BULLY: I don't have any friends and I'm always in trouble at school.
DONNA: What's your family like?
MITCH AS BULLY: They're divorced. My mom works nights and I never see my dad anymore. I'm alone a lot.

In other sessions with Mitch in which discipline was required in actual situations that arose, we would have him play the parent who would mete out some reaction to "his son's" bad behavior. Still in the role of the parent, we would have him explain his rationale for the disciplinary action. Invariably, Mitch would learn something more about himself and some of the rules of life in our family. My wife and I would also benefit from these sessions by learning something more about how he perceived us and what his *real and deeper reactions* were to our behavior.

Children do not usually answer *direct* questions. Role-playing can often provide useful information to a parent that can later be of benefit to the child. For example, when we would get curious about Mitch's situation at school, we would have him play the role of his teacher and then ask: "Mrs. Smith, how's Mitch doing in class?"

MITCH AS MRS. SMITH: "He's a great reader, but he's not too good in math, and sometimes he fools around too much. But he's a fine boy and I like him."

On other occasions, we would get reports that were not as salutary.

The use of role-playing can be effective in the general socialization of a child. A psychodrama student of mine presented the following report on her use of role-playing with her child.

When my child is smacking his lips, eating sloppily or displaying poor manners, role-playing, especially role-reversal, offers an excellent means of making a point without nagging or spoiling an otherwise good situation. The parent can merely mimic the child's displeasing or inappropriate behavior and, as the child looks on, the point is rapidly driven home. The child can then alter his behavior without undue embarrassment to himself or being subjected to parental nagging.

This particular technique has worked well with my son, George. Recently, when he was ill and had to take some medicine, I assumed his role and jumped up and down and carried on as he was doing over some medicine he was being asked to take. I was amazed at how suddenly his behavior ceased, and he quietly followed me into the kitchen for a spoon to take the medicine. Somehow the sight of his mother jumping up and down, stomping her feet, and carrying on had a very sobering effect on George. I have also applied this technique successfully to correct sloppy eating habits in George. I merely smack my lips, eat and chew loudly, and generally mimic his behavior and I see immediate improvement after first watching a blush of embarrassment cross his face.

I also find role reversal is a very successful technique to use to draw my son out when he is reluctant to open up with the details of a "bad" day, the problems he is experiencing at school, or how he thinks his teacher feels about him. His day-to-day behavior serves as a clue to me that things are not going well and it is time to use some psychodrama and get at the real problems that are bugging him. I recently missed a good opportunity to use the method to help my son talk about a scary situation in which he was bitten by a large German shepherd. I could have assumed the role of the dog and encouraged George to talk to the dog about how he felt about his biting him, then I could have had George play the dog and I could have been George.

I recently applied role reversal to an impasse my son and I had reached over whether he would continue to study his spelling words. I called for a role reversal, and as George, I proceeded to balk and refuse to spell my words. George as me was quick to pick up my nagging approach, and then reinforced it with a doubled-up fist placed at eye level. He then said, "If you don't spell those words, I'm going to punch you in the nose and stomach." I suddenly realized that this was my son's projection of how his mother was treating him. I later confirmed my fear by relating the experience to my therapist, who said yes, I do tend to resort to a show of force and often unfairly use my position of authority. I have tried to correct this tendency on my part.

Zerka Moreno performed many impromptu acts of psychodrama with her son Jonathan when he was a young child that are useful in other impromptu situations. Among the many dialogues found in J. L., Zerka, and Jonathan Moreno's book, *The First Psychodramatic Family* is the following use of role reversal "at home":

> Mother says to Jonathan, "Eat—eat—eat!"
> Jonathan is annoyed and says to himself,
> "But why?—I'm not hungry."

> Mother says to Jonathan, "Finish the meal,
> You have so much on the plate."
> Jonathan thinks, "Why should I finish
> If I don't feel like it?"
> Mother thinks he looks pale,
> He had the flu, and lost weight.
> Jonathan cries.

> Mother says, "Let's reverse roles."
> Jonathan in the role of mother:
> "Eat, eat everything on your plate,
> You can't leave the table yet
> Because you are not through."
> Mother as Jonathan:
> "But I am full. I can't take another bite."
> Jonathan as mother calmly replies:
> "So don't eat!"

> Jonathan becomes himself
> And returns to his seat.
> Mother returns to her seat deeply impressed

And says:
"Jonathan, eat only as much as you want
And when you are through you can leave the table."
Here Jonathan is not only his own therapist,
But the therapist of his mother as well.*

In this pattern of role-playing sessions with children, a psycho-drama student of mine, Joe Lamontagne, developed what might be termed psychodramatic family fantasy games. In a report to me on this creation, Lamontagne wrote that he based the games on the following premise about psychodrama and children:

> Children love to play-act. They love to fantasize. Their level of spontaneity is clearly the least corrupted by our society's hideous version of social adaptation. Not surprisingly, very few and very limited modifications are required to effect the transition between psychodrama sessions, which produce new responses to old situations or generate adequate responses to new ones, and fantasy encounter games. Psychodrama synthesizes childlike fantasies into dramatic situations where they can be recognized, enacted, and infused into day-to-day activity.

Joe played around twenty rounds of psychodrama games with his wife and four daughters, aged five, seven, eleven, and twelve. The children were apparently most responsive, especially the seven- and eleven-year-old girls. After dinner, the family, on a scheduled basis, ignored the TV culture-conserve that formerly dominated their lives and set aside two to three hours for their sessions. The "protagonist" would select an area of interest from a list of twenty topics and then begin to have a session using role-reversal, doubles, soliloquy, and other psychodramatic techniques. The list included the following topics or games:

> Tell your father (or mother) what you would do differently if you were in his (her) place. Why? (If you're a parent, tell your child.)
> Think about one person or thing that makes you angry. Tell your partner what you really think about it, what you're going to

* J. L., Zerka and Jonathan Moreno, *The First Psychodramatic Family* (New York: Beacon House, 1964), pp. 81–82.

do about it. What have you already done? Did it help? Why, or why not? This would invariably lead into a situation, such as an incident at school, work, or at the playground.

You are a new person in a group. In order to join, you must explain to the other members why they should want you as a member, and answer any questions they may have. Here the family would play the role of the new group as defined by the "potential member," and ask probing questions about his character.

Is there someone whom you are afraid of for any reason? Your partner will be that person for the next few minutes. Discuss that fear, and see what both of you can do about it.

What would the *perfect* world be like? How would it look? Where would it be? Who would be in it? What would be the most important thing about it?

As far as you can tell, what do people think of you? Become some other person, and tell your partner all about your (real) self, as you think others see you. How important is it to you whether others like you? Why, or why not?

My student indicated that his children especially enjoyed and benefited from the game related to telling your mother or father what you would do differently if you were in his or her place:

One by one, each child really laid into her father. Then we did a role-reversal, and *I* had a go at that tyrant (me), despite some very sound arguments from the old man (age 11) about parental responsibility. Then we reversed back to our own roles, and I caught it in unison, a cappella, fortissimo. That session both awakened me to my weakness as the local patriarch and I think let them—for the first time—fully believe that honest expression was not only tolerated in this family milieu but encouraged.

Psychodramas related to a person's work are useful and meaningful sessions. As a standard session, have a protagonist ask for a raise, then reverse roles and become his own boss. In the role of the boss, the protagonist should either give the raise or not, and then go into detail about the reason for the positive or negative decision. Members of the group should ask the protagonist in the role of his boss pointed questions about his employee, such as his strong and weak points. Another universal type of session related to the work role is to project the protagonist ten years into the future and have him psychodramatically enact the position he will then have and how he likes it.

A dress salesman who participated in a number of psychodramas told me how he improvised a psychodramatic method *in situ* that has effectively helped him in his work and as a side effect enlarged his income. "After I show my dress line, without warning I reverse roles by doubling for the buyer and voice all of her objections to the line and what she's thinking. Even when I'm only half right, the buyer gets such a kick out of my act that she buys more than she ordinarily would. The technique loosens up the buyer and improves our communication."

Religious psychodramas are often complex but produce intriguing sessions. Have a person play the role of his God. The group should provoke "God" to state as many details about His (or Her) meaning as possible. When projected into the role of their next life, people have fascinating responses. Some people have concrete concepts of heaven and hell and how they will wind up. Others have very hazy concepts, if any, about where or what they will be beyond this life. The enigma of the ultimate role of being dead that confronts everyone can be usefully explored in a psychodrama group.

Impromptu sessions between spouses are often useful. My wife, Donna, and I often reverse roles on the spot when conflict emerges. Sometimes a simple role reversal can resolve a complex problem. Seeing the situation from the perspective of the other (if you really get into it) can be a useful device.

Another impromptu psychodramatic method that is functional is the future-projection technique. When you have an important meeting coming up, or are about to make a crucial phone call, it is often valuable to act it out in advance, with a friend in the role of the other. Invariably, the session will provide new insights and information of value—and you improve your effectiveness in the real situation. It tends to make your performance more effective in the situation, since you have already "been there."

A psychodrama exercise I would recommend for *everyone* could be entitled "How to become your own best psychodramatist" or *"exploring your social atom."* The exercise can be enacted alone or in the presence of one or more people close to you. If someone else is present, they can double for you or remain silent.

The first step in "exploring your social atom" is to draw a sociogram of your social atom with *you* at the center as the nucleus. Before you draw your sociogram, think about and list the significant people in your life. By significant, I mean people who are emotionally important to you. In most cases, these will be people you love, but significance can also encompass a complex hate-love and even guilt relationship. Consider the emotional distance that exists between you and the three, four, or five most significant people in your life. (Do not, ordinarily, consider more than five people, since it becomes too complex.) For example, the following sociogram reveals my social atom and the emotional distance between me and the significant people in my life—at least at this time. (It is important to note that some people have a relatively constant permanent social atom, whereas some people's social atoms change periodically. This factor is a useful self-diagnostic factor.)

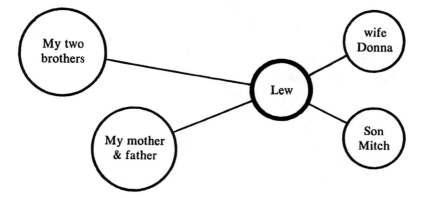

In drawing my personal sociogram, I immediately became aware of the fact that my wife and son are closest to me and almost equidistant emotionally. Also I note that *my* mother and father and my brothers are paired in distance.

There are many complexities to a social atom. For some people, *one* person may be clearly the one and only closest person. In other atoms, there are several people in the same social-emotional position vis-à-vis you.

In some cases, a person who is deceased is very important, sometimes more important than anyone alive. A married man's mistress may be emotionally closer to him than his wife. A child may, almost symbiotically, be in a person's own circle—this is, of course, psychologically and physically true for a woman when she is pregnant. When a married couple's circles intersect, this closeness can be positive or negative. It can reflect a positive emotional closeness or a pathological symbiotic dependency relationship. It is up to the people involved to determine this. Everyone's social atom is unique and distinctive. Simply drawing it, then studying it, can begin to set off emotional waves and provide significant insights.

After you have drawn and *studied* your social atom, act it out. This is done by placing your "self" in a chair and placing your "others" as empty chairs around you. Take the role of each person in your social atom in turn. I would suggest allocating around five or ten minutes for each performance of the people in your atom. The chair can be occupied by "you" in the role of the other if you are alone, or someone can be an auxiliary ego, take the role of the "other," and talk back.

You can say anything you want to your "self" in the role of the other in the chair. For example, in one case, a wife playing her husband covered the following issues: (1) the quality of their sex life—what "he" liked and didn't like about her performance; (2) whether "he" planned to spend his life with her or not; (3) the things about her that annoyed him the most, and the things about her he liked best; (4) "his" judgment about her in the role of mother; (5) a review of her sexual fidelity, or lack thereof; and (6) "his" judgment of her "mental health."

The same woman played the role of her son and in the role of her son discussed the following issues in response to an auxiliary

ego playing her: (1) whether or not "his" mother was a just dis-
ciplinarian; (2) the things "he" liked most and least about "his"
mother; (3) whether or not "his" mother gave "him" enough attention; and (4) did she really want "him" when "he" was born.

Playing the role of the relevant others in your social atom has
parallels to the physical health checkup that everyone periodically
requires. In this case, the enactment of your social atom provides
the opportunity for a necessary emotional checkup. If you and
everyone in your social atom did this regularly, it could help revolve problems, reduce conflict, and make for a fuller, happier life
situation.

In all of the approaches described, psychodrama becomes a
valuable rehearsal for life. It also is useful for enlarging the scope
of a person's perspective by providing the opportunity to play
more varied roles. No doubt, as you, your family, or your impromptu group act out the exercises suggested here, you will
spontaneously go off into other arenas, and this is a desirable
consequence. The models presented here are only preliminary
suggestions, and hopefully they will spark the group to a variety
of spontaneous and creative sessions. Psychodrama is most effective with a trained psychodramatist in a group setting, but its
impromptu uses outside of a formal construct can become a
valuable adjunct to resolving problems of everyday life and enlarging your social perspective.

Psychodrama for a Mass Audience

Psychodramatic performances, like theatrical performances in the
mass media, can be geared for a wider mass audience than the
people present in an immediate small group and can encompass
and affect a wider audience than the personal problems of the people immediately present at a session. Sessions with a mass audience
can take at least three forms: (1) the session can be run directly

with a large group; (2) a small group of from fifteen to twenty people can be invited on stage and a session can be run with the small group in front of the larger group; or (3) a session can be directed with a small group in a studio—filmed or videotaped—and projected to a mass audience.

The living newspaper is a type of psychodrama for a mass audience. In this form, the fear and anxiety about large, generally uncontrollable events of cataclysmic proportions to the average person—such as assassinations, war, earthquakes, and crime—can be reduced in people's lives through psychodrama. Moreno's early research with the relationships between theatrical performances and the realities of "life" were illuminating experiences. In particular, his invention of "the living newspaper" brought to life relatively flat events presented in the press, and this enabled people to better comprehend the meaning of these events in their life. In an article in the *New York Sun* (March 30, 1931), a reporter summarized Moreno's concept of the "living newspaper": "The audience at the Guild Theater on Sunday will see a 'newsreel' of current events created in stage form under their very noses, acted without any sort of rehearsal. It will be possible to read in the *Sun* on Saturday evening the account of a bank robbery, a public ceremony or the death of a prominent man and to see that selfsame incident portrayed on the stage only twenty-four hours later."

During my work with Dr. Moreno, I participated in a variety of "living newspaper" events. For example, in 1961, Adolf Eichmann was on trial in Israel. The trial had a profound and powerful impact on many people all over the world and especially in the United States. Those who had a personal relationship to the atrocities of Nazism were most deeply affected by the trial of this Nazi executioner, but almost everyone had a reaction to the event.

For these reasons, Dr. Moreno ran a mass psychodrama at the American Psychiatric Association Meeting in Chicago in May of 1961. There were about three hundred people present at Moreno's session. At Dr. Moreno's request, I reluctantly agreed to play the role of the despised Adolf Eichmann. I psyched myself up for the part by reading everything I could on Eichmann's "I was only following orders" defense (a defense that has since acquired a certain universal quality; e.g., the Watergate conspirators and Lt. William Calley's defense for My Lai).

The session began with a group warm-up discussion. Moreno called me forward and placed me on a high stage in the center of the group. He then introduced me as Adolf Eichmann. A fellow psychodramatist, Dr. Richard Korn, played the role of Israel's chief prosecuting attorney.

I plunged into the role, defending myself as a man following orders who would have certainly been killed by Adolf Hitler if I didn't carry out his mandate to exterminate the Jews and other political enemies of Germany. "What about my family?" I implored of the group. "We had to survive."

The results were electrifying during the entire three hours of the session. Many psychiatrists in the group were refugees from Germany and had lost members of their family in the death camps administered by Eichmann. Although it was only a psychodramatic living newspaper, it became immediate and emotional to everyone present. People rose up in tears and began to vilify me in the role of Eichmann with horrendous curses and denunciations.

The central impacts of the session were a profound catharsis for the group and the articulation of deeper feelings about the catastrophe that until this enactment lay festering in the participant's psyche. Many people in the group "found each other," cried together, and discussed a psychic pain that was formerly felt in loneliness and despair prior to the session. Many people embraced, and the group of several hundred developed a marvelous cohesion and empathy.

The session provided the opportunity for the group to personally explore in a group psychodrama the agony each felt privately on encountering this formerly devastating impersonal world event. The warm and affectionate results of the session were clearly manifest in the group.

My only reward for playing the role of Eichmann was a greater understanding of his psychopathic mind because there was a carry-over of hostility toward me for playing the role. That night at dinner and the next morning at breakfast many people (some unconsciously) glowered at me—as the arch-villain Eichmann. It took some time before several people could respond to me as nice-guy colleague Lew Yablonsky.

In another mass psychodrama session of this type, Moreno produced The Psychodrama of the Assassination of John F. Kennedy at the American Psychiatric Association meeting in Los Angeles in June 1964. For this session he asked me to play Lee Harvey Oswald. Recalling my Eichmann experience, I refused and acquired the somewhat more sympathetic role of Jack Ruby. Dr. George Bach, an eminent psychologist and longtime associate of Moreno and mine, played the role of Oswald. Enormous sympathy was generated for Zerka Moreno, who played Jackie Kennedy. Donna Yablonsky, in the role of one of the members of the jury that tried Jack Ruby, synthesized the sense of anguish and despair felt by the over five hundred people present at the session.

Many members of the group later told me that the session clarified and catharted many painful emotions they had held in since the actual assassination. They felt relieved to express their feelings and in the process experienced a sense of relief of their pain when they became aware of the fact that thousands—no doubt millions—of other people shared their emotions.

There is great value in the psychodramatic production of significant events for a large group. The nature of the mass media tends to depersonalize events that have great meaning to people on a very personal level. Television and films constantly bombard people with the horrendous events of war, homicide, famine, and accidents. A general reaction is to repress the deep emotional feelings of helplessness and frustration generated about these events. A mass psychodrama session enables people to present their formerly bottled-up emotions about these happenings, articulate the size and shape of their real feelings, and in some measure achieve a degree of beneficial catharsis.

Beyond the confines of a session with an immediate large group, there has been some experimentation with projecting a group psychodrama about specific personal problems through television and films to a mass audience. The results have been generally excellent, although there are some complex problems in the process that require solution.

Over the years I have directed a number of psychodrama sessions that were videotaped or filmed and later projected to a mass audience. In one network television production I helped produce, I directed over fifty hours of psychodrama in a television studio with a "repertory" group of people randomly cast from the community who presented their own personal dramas. The group was composed of a cross-section of people recruited for the show, including old, young, black, brown, and white, with varying political positions. All of the sessions were videotaped and the peak sessions were edited and utilized for the various themes of the series. The results were shown in twelve programs on 226 Public Broadcasting System stations around the country.

The sessions were slices of Americana and included: a black woman whose militant activities against racism and the oppression of women produced complex family problems; an articulate and creative man in a robot job who felt he had wasted his life; a poor gas station attendant who fervently believed in and defended a society that had obviously given him the short end; a young black man who believed on a deep level that the death of his "Uncle Tom" father would liberate him and his own son; a young woman who vacillated and commuted between a hip, communal life and a "straight" existence; a young man into gay liberation who was having "marital problems" with his wife, Bill; and other, more standard lifestyle problems.

The sessions had some parallels to a version of "psychodrama" presented in Shakespeare's *Hamlet*. Everyone who has read *Hamlet* recalls the marvelous situation in which Hamlet, with the aid of a traveling band of actors, stages a scene to get a reaction from his errant and guilty mother. In this Shakespeare psychodrama, they reproduce the real-life event where the new king (Hamlet's uncle) kills Hamlet's father as he sleeps in the palace garden and then marries the queen—Hamlet's mother. The impact of this vile deed performed in the psychodrama-like scene before the king, and queen, and their court was the climax of the play. One difference among many between this Shakspearean dramatic use of role-playing and contemporary psychodrama is that in psychodrama Hamlet plays Hamlet.

As in Shakespeare, it was hoped that the "court," in our TV psychodrama community-viewing audience, would benefit from seeing something of their own drama or that of their "brothers" and "sisters" portrayed in depth. One assumption of the program was that there was a greater potential for personal identification with a real person acting out his own drama than with an actor in a fictional play. This mass media vehicle attempted to produce sessions that would have enough impact on a mass audience so that they might gain some insights into their personal and emotional existence, even though they were not physically present at the actual session.

The viewing audience's involvement was, in great measure, contingent on how much personal truth the psychodramatic protagonist could convey to the mass audience of millions of people. The sessions seemed to reach some deep levels of human experience and had an impact on many people beyond the immediate group. This was evidenced by the audience response in thousands of letters that indicated a personal identification with the problems and conflicts presented on television. The program also received positive critical reviews on this perspective of mass impact from over a hundred sources. Several specific critics (in addition to many others) analyzed and reflected a positive response to the intent and meaning of the programs:

> *Psychodramas:* "The Family Game" offers an entirely different family line. The twelve-week series, produced by WQED in Pittsburgh for the Public Broadcasting Service's network of 226 stations, presents real parents and children in a taped, group-encounter session, in the hope that viewers will apply the psychodramas to their own problems. Guided by sociologist Lewis

Yablonsky, participants act out their most intense feelings about freedom and authority, sex, drugs and race prejudice.

On a recent segment, a middle-aged gas-station manager named Tony angrily tangled with several counterculturists in the group. "You need mental treatment!" he exploded after learning that a young girl panelist was shacking up in a commune. Another searing moment came when a troubled young black pointed an imaginary gun at his middle-class father and spewed out a lifetime of loathing for the way his father was "playin' whitey's game." At the close of each show, the leader urges viewers to adapt the discussions to their own hangups.

—Newsweek, November 6, 1972

. . . a young black man, encounters his own despair. He rages against his father for allowing white society to humiliate him. He rages against that society for forcing his father, and him, to play its game. And he rages at the knowledge that it will do the same to his son. With the help of another participant, he acts out a confrontation with his father in which he threatens to kill him. He affirms violent revolt. "A pistol puts you in charge." And through it all, he cries.

It is a rage and a pain black people—particularly black people with children—must deal with somehow. But it is not a parlor game. Even with the gently controlling presence of master psychodramatist, Dr. Lewis Yablonsky, the reassuring social director of the psyche who set up these episodes, George's responses are personally explosive.

—The New York Times
Sunday, October 1, 1972

Accustomed to stagnant spectator roles before the big eye in the living room, we've gone a long way toward losing the art of conversation and, more particularly, the art of communicating meaningfully with each other.

"The Family Game" hopes to start us on the way back. Subtitled "Identities for Young and Old," the half-hour programs enable us to watch real people—not movie stars—act out their feelings on subjects that touch their daily lives.

There is real drama here. It is not soap suds.

The series deals realistically with fathers and sons, drugs, sex, religion, what real patriotism is, and other gut issues troubling us today in all our homes.

Courier Express
October 10, 1972 (Buffalo, New York)

The Marriage Game

Based on our success with psychodrama on *The Family Game,* I developed another type of TV program that would focus more precisely on marital problems and issues. The following treatment of this type of program delineates some of the issues and impacts of doing psychodrama on TV.

On *The Marriage Game,* average people with relatively normal marriage problems would act out their conflicts in psychodrama with auxiliary egos assuming the role of their spouses. The program would open on nine people (including myself) seated in a semicircle discussing the problems of marriage in contemporary society. In front of the group would be a stage, set as a combination bedroom-living room. It is apparent that a drama will soon unfold onstage. The discussion and the camera begins to reveal who the nine people are, as in turn we would introduce ourselves. The group would be comprised of myself, two trained auxiliary egos, and two married couples who were experiencing conflict. As the program began, I would rapidly focus the married couples on a problem they are experiencing.

The session takes place in a large studio, and there are several types of "audiences" participating in the session: (1) the group of eight immediate participants in my psychodrama session; (2) a studio audience of several hundred people, preferably married couples, watching the psychodrama; and (3) the mass audience of several million people who would see the show on television.

Example Session. The following dialogue and description is derived from a session I have actually directed. It reflects the type of session that could spontaneously emerge in a TV program on marriage. Moreover, based on many sessions I have directed, it reflects a common marital problem in contemporary society.

MONICA: My whole life revolves around him and the children. There is no Monica, only Jack and his wife. I have to get out of this or go mad. I'm depressed most of the time. Now on top of all this *HE* wants an open marriage so HE can go out and screw some young chippie without guilt.

JACK: She's exaggerating. I do everything I can to be a good husband to her—but someone has to take care of the house. And about the open marriage thing. We're into a new period of sexual openness in the seventies and frankly after fifteen years, she bores me in bed.

L.Y.: Monica, when do you argue about these issues?

MONICA: Usually around bedtime, after the kids are sleeping. It's the only time I see him anymore.

L.Y.: Okay, Monica—come on up on the stage. An auxiliary ego will play your husband.

After Monica sets the scene with her husband, Jack, they begin to discuss their life together. As the session unfolds, it becomes apparent that she has begun to hate him, because she feels she is totally dependent on him.

She reverses roles and plays her husband. In his role, she expresses how she believes he feels about her now.

MONICA AS JACK: I'm sick of you—you're a terrible pain in the ass. If there was a way out—without losing my kids and everything I've worked for—I'd leave immediately.

L.Y. (to the real Jack, seated near the stage): How do you feel about what she said as you?

JACK: I still love her—but I guess she doesn't know that. Maybe I never tell her anymore.

MONICA: He's a goddamn liar. I'm furious with him.

L.Y.: Have you ever felt like hitting him?

MONICA: Plenty of times, but I never have because that would be the end of our marriage.

I hand Monica a battoca.

L.Y.: Set up a scene in which you really get mad at him. You can hit him here with no penalty. Is that okay with you, Jack? (I turn to the real Jack.)

JACK (*with a forced smile on his face*): Sure. Let's get it on.

We cut back to stage. "Jack" begins to tell her how she's just a little girl who couldn't do anything in the real world anyway: "Without me, you're nothing," etc.

Monica blows up in tears and anger and begins to hit "Jack" with the battoca. It begins to feel good to her, as she catharts her hostility.

L.Y.: Now I want you to hit him—only each time say what it's for.
HIT
MONICA: That's for making me feel like I'm nothing.
HIT
MONICA: That's for not spending enough time with me and the kids.
HIT
MONICA: That's for not really wanting me anymore.
> *Monica continues with her aggression, then breaks into tears. She looks at the real Jack, smiles through her tears, and says: "You know, you son-of-a-bitch, in spite of this I still really love you!"*
L.Y.: When did you love him the most?
MONICA: When we were first married.
> *Now that her hostility has been somewhat ventilated, we go back in time. I set up the scene of their marriage ceremony. "Jack" and Monica stand before the minister* (played by one of the psychodrama assistants).
L.Y.: Here you are twenty-two and marrying Jack. Soliloquize (à la Hamlet) your thoughts as the ceremony is going on.
MONICA: Here I am—fat Monica—and I've caught a beautiful man. I'm ecstatic. Everything I ever wanted is going to happen for me. I'll never let him down. We'll have beautiful children, and life will be wonderful.
> *In this scene we had the real Jack come forward and alongside of the actor soliloquize* his *hopes and feelings at the time of his marriage.*
L.Y.: Here you are today, Monica, after fifteen years, despondent, wanting out of the marriage. What happened?

Monica begins to talk about how society is different today, how she is now part of a weekly woman's consciousness-raising group and she feels that she should be more of a total person than she is, that she expects more from her husband. Here we did a five-minute scene with Monica in her group, and another scene with Monica playing her mother delineating how a wife should be from her viewpoint.

L.Y.: Now that we have seen something of Monica's perception of the marriage, let's have the real Jack come up on the psychodrama stage to present his side of the marriage.

Jack comes up and we have Monica, played by an auxiliary ego, appear on stage with him. He goes through several scenes that depict his marital emotions. He is bored with their sex and manifests a degree of impotency with his wife, but not with other women. At forty, he feels he has achieved only a few of his lifetime aspirations. When his wife nags him, she reminds him of his mother, toward whom we find he has great hostility.

At this point, the group is involved and all members of the psychodrama cast discuss various meanings and implications of the session. One auxiliary ego says, "I wasn't acting in that one scene—when I was Monica and wanted to work and have my own identity. When I was married, that was my exact problem. This session reminded me of that time and I'm resolved never to get into that bind again."

(If this session had been done in the studio I described earlier, I would at this point have opened up the session to the points of emotional identification felt by the larger group present. As the director of the session, I would have begun to elicit their responses to the psychodrama, *NOT* as analysts, but relating their personal lives to the experience.)

In the actual session with Monica and Jack, I had Monica play a final scene, one that never happened in her real life. I place her in a lawyer's office, setting up her divorce. In this part of the session, I had her enact two possible scenes of resolution.

POSSIBLE SCENE I (*summarized conclusion*):
LAWYER: Well, now that you've told me all the reasons for your wanting a divorce, just sign here and you're free.
MONICA: Fine (She signs.)
LAWYER: How do you feel?
MONICA: I'm a little sad, but I have a bright new life in my future.

POSSIBLE SCENE II:
LAWYER: Well, now that you've told me all the reasons for your wanting a divorce, just sign here and you're free.

MONICA (breaks into tears): I can't do this. I love Jack, my children, and our life together.

The real Jack comes on stage. They embrace.

JACK: Darling, I love you. I'm glad we finally got all of this out. We'll work at it and have the beautiful life together we deserve.

This was, in fact, the conclusion to Jack and Monica's session. The group present responded in a variety of ways. Some indicated how they had a "therapeutic divorce," others agreed they should continue to work at the marriage.

Of the three groups delineated earlier, who would be "participants" in the session, there is a degree of predictability about the positive emotional meaning of the session to the two groups physically present. With regard to the mass audience, viewing the session on a TV screen, there is not enough experience to come to any definitive conclusion about the impact of psychodrama. Many people, however, who viewed the P.B.S. *Family Game* did write in to the effect that the sessions stimulated productive family encounters and discussions.

There are other kinds of problems and issues related to doing psychodrama in the mass media. One is that in any psychodrama session, whether in a small theater or on national TV, there is an impact not only on the people present but on the people to whom the protagonists are directly related. For example, if a wife has a session in the studio, it is found to eventually affect her parents, husband, and children in some way when they see the session. What she expresses about her family has impact and consequences.

In any session, therefore, there is a necessary concern with the people not present who are portrayed by members of the group. For example, one young man in his twenties had a blockbuster psychodrama session filmed in the TV studio of *The Family Game*, but it was never broadcast for various reasons. In the session, he unleashed his enormous hostility toward his father. His venom was so strong that in a scene where he was "punching" his father psychodramatically, he broke a foam-rubber board that we used to symbolically represent his father's face. He later role-reversed and played his father, a high school principal and a right-wing political extremist who would get drunk and beat up him and his mother for no apparent reason. The young man, in psychodrama, revealed his personal portrait of Dad. We saw the sharp image of a father who was overtly a Mr. American-Good Guy; and hypocritically, on another level, a man tragically seething with venom that he acted out behind closed doors on his family. The program depicted a negative image of "Dad" that went far beyond any depicted on television so far—including Archie Bunker.

Based on other psychodrama sessions I have directed, I know that this type of person is an American prototype. As such, in my view this image should have been exposed on TV, if only to equalize and give the other version of "Dad." Not all Dads are understanding, like Robert Young's *Father Knows Best* and Fred McMurray's apple pie father image in *My Three Sons*. This other type of "Dad" could have been seen for perhaps the first time on TV in the context of psychodrama. The session, no doubt, could have had some definite effect on this actual father as well as on the mass audience of fathers and sons viewing the session in their homes. These images of "Dad" have certainly been portrayed in fictionalized dramas, but with psychodrama the viewing audience would have known they are real people and the impact would have been different—possibly more emotionally potent.

Psychodrama has enormous impact on all groups observing a session, and it is almost impossible to be a dispassionate observer. Everyone tends to become a participant rather than a voyeur because he hears, sees, and feels certain important dimensions of his own life in action. Audiences have an enormous curiosity and interest in observing the emotional experiences of others—especially when the portrayal goes beyond the superficial. In this context, psychodrama is one of the most exciting and fascinating vehicles for presenting the inner life of people to a vast audience, because psychodrama involves real people enacting their actual life dramas.

Producing psychodramas on film for a mass audience is still in the experimental stage of development; yet we have proven that psychodrama can be enacted in a studio with effective theatrical devices of lighting and sets. The program can then be shown to millions of people who can experience the psychodrama session on their own home set in the company of their friends and family. Psychodrama as theater, for a mass audience, may eventually be the medium that will most successfully convey its potentially powerful humanistic effect on people. This impact may be emotionally more potent than theater because psychodrama has an existential validity and reality quite different from theater.

CHAPTER

6

Psychodrama: Theater and Life

Imagine that you have received some insult in public, perhaps a slap in the face, that makes your cheek burn whenever you think of it. The inner shock was so great that it blotted out all the details of this harsh incident. But some insignificant thing will instantly revive the memory of the insult, and the emotion will recur with redoubled violence. Your cheek will grow red or you will turn pale and your heart will pound.

If you possess such sharp and easily aroused emotional material you will find it easy to transfer it to the stage and play a scene analogous to the experience you had in real life which left such a shocking impression on you. To do this you will not need any technique. It will play itself because nature will help you.

—Constantin Stanislavski,
An Actor Prepares *

* Constantin Stanislavski, *An Actor Prepares* (New York: Theatre Arts Books, 1969), p. 176.

To bid us, as Shaw, Wilde, Yeats, and
Santayana do, find the splendid mask,
or the appropriate one, is counsel of
perfection. Most of us are condemned,
by "life" or by ourselves, to fig leaf—
or inadequate mask. We do not live
well. Life is a drama; but we cannot
play our role properly.
—Eric Bentley,
The Life of the Drama †

MARLON BRANDO, when flattered by Dick Cavett on a
talk show as "one of the greatest actors of our time," demurred:
"Everybody is an actor. You're doing it now. You are playing
the role of an interviewer. People play the roles of parents, politicians, teachers. Everyone is a natural actor."

Of course, in one sense Brando is correct. Everyone must learn
to act in order to participate in life. It is apparent that until one
reclines at night, one is role-playing—enacting various motives,
attitudes, and postures. Not only theatrical actors, therefore, but
everyone gives a variety of performances every day of his life.

The intellectual exercise of relating everyday life performance
to life on a theatrical stage has preoccupied many philosophers
and dramatists. Among others, Stanislavsky, in his classic *An
Actor Prepares,* was one of the first to detail the application of personal moods and emotions to theatrical performance. Although
Stanislavsky encouraged spontaneity and improvisation on the part
of the actor, the Stanislavsky approach to acting is distinctly different from psychodrama in at least one major respect. The Stanislavsky method calls for the use of emotion and experiences to perfect
the actor's ability in a *theatrical role.* Psychodrama, in contrast,
utilizes a person's emotions and experiences for the basic goal of
improving his performance *in life.* Moreover, in psychodrama the
immediate experience of the session has personal value; whereas

† Eric Bentley, *The Life of the Drama* (New York: Atheneum, 1967),
p. 185.

the Stanislavsky method is a training process for some future theatrical performance.

In a reverse context, in theorizing about human behavior, sociologist Erving Goffman, in his book *The Presentation of Self in Everyday Life,* describes the manner in which "performances" in everyday life have "dramaturgical" implications.

> The perspective employed in this report is that of the theatrical performance; the principles derived are dramaturgical ones. I shall consider the way in which the individual in ordinary work situations presents himself and his activity to others, the ways in which he guides and controls the impression they form of him, and the kinds of things he may and may not do while sustaining his performance before them. In using this model I will attempt not to make light of its obvious inadequacies. The stage presents things that are make-believe; presumably life presents things that are real and sometimes not well rehearsed. More important, perhaps, on the stage one player presents himself in the guise of a character to characters projected by other players; the audience constitutes a third party to the interaction—one that is essential and yet, if the stage performance were real, one that would not be there. In real life, the three parties are compressed into two; the part one individual plays is tailored to the parts played by the others present, and yet these others also constitute the audience. . . .*

Goffman's goal for his model is essentially to utilize the dramaturgical conceptual scheme for understanding behavior. His analysis is geared toward the laudable goal of comprehending human performance with greater clarity. Certainly psychodrama as "a mirror of life" also achieves this goal—perhaps with greater control and in greater depth—but psychodrama has the additional dimensions of effectively modifying behavior in more personally satisfying and productive directions.

Eric Bentley, a literary critic and professor of drama, spent a considerable amount of time studying the relationship of life to drama. In his play *Are You Now Or Have You Ever Been* he

* Erving Goffman, *The Presentation of Self in Everyday Life* (New York: Doubleday, Anchor Books, 1959), p. xi.

extracts the actual dialogue of the political witch hunts of the fifties and artistically presents brilliant theater. In one of his books, *The Life of the Drama,* he makes a cogent appraisal of the relationship of psychodrama to theater and its meaning to everyday life:

> . . . doctors, especially those of certain schools, have observed and accepted the human tendency to take this world as a theatre. In Freudian psychoanalysis, the therapist is assigned all the co-starring roles by the patient, who is of course the star, and a grand re-enactment of childhood scenes takes place, five acts a week for as long as neurosis, or money, or patience lasts.
>
> One celebrated therapist, J. L. Moreno, objects to the Freudian procedure on the grounds (if I may paraphrase him) that it is not nearly theatrical enough. "The mind is a stage," one reporter on Moreno's procedure has said. Moreno finds the silent, unseen, note-taking man behind the couch too undramatic; likewise, the talkative fellow on the couch, his eyes on the ceiling, saying all the things he daren't say into anyone's face. Life is a successful piece of theatre in which people sit and stand as they will, in which dialogue is reciprocal, in which people gesticulate *at* each other, and look each other in the eye, whether from interest, affection or dislike. Living is to exist with all these means of direct personal communication working spontaneously. Neurosis, or failing to live, is to exist without such spontaneity, with fears and hates that interfere so much that (at an extreme) one either runs away from the other person or assaults him. Moreno accordingly argues that no cure can be attempted without making the patient work directly on the drama he wishes to live. How is that possible? A drama has a number of characters in it. What about the others beside the patient? Moreno appeals to the principle of theatre itself: substitution of one person for another, role playing. The therapist is assigned roles, not merely, as in Freudian procedure, in the patient's imagination, but physically, upon a stage. Auxiliary therapists take stage to fill other parts. The patient has to confront them, and not in reconstruction of the past only, as in the reconstructions of crimes by the police, but in scenes arising newly and now. All this (to complete the theatrical circuit) with other patients watching, i.e., unshielded from "the others," taking place in society, in the world.
>
> The instinctive reaction of each of us is: "*I* could never do

that, I'd sink through the floor!" But it has been found that people, after a "warming up" period, can "do that," and that there is no great problem about getting people's family dramas enacted, spontaneously and vigorously, upon Dr. Moreno's "psychodramatic" stage. What therapeutic success has been attained by the method is not the question here, nor shall I go into Moreno's preference for his "real" dramas to the dramas written by playwrights. I have set down this description of what I understand psychodrama to be because it offers the most vivid evidence imaginable of the intimate link between theatre and life. Even if the therapeutic results were small, one could scarcely doubt that Moreno is "on to" something. Schopenhauer always maintained that "the drama is the most perfect reflection of human existence" and I must confess I had always read that sentence as a bit of magniloquence until it was made real for me by a reading of Moreno.*

Psychodrama has values of its own, but I would not dispute Bentley's assessment that psychodrama is also magnificent theater. We can see some of the relationships between theater and psychodrama; however, a more complex question relates to the differences and similarities between these forms of human behavior and everyday life.

There are many nuances of difference between theatrical acting and performance in everyday life. One, as indicated, is that most people are enacting their personal lives and postures in relatively spontaneous situations, without prescribed specific lines even thought the cultural norms do require a generally expected response. In contrast, a theatrical performer tends to have lines and movements usually written and directed by someone else.

Role-enactment in the theater, therefore, is a form peculiarly different from acting in everyday life. Actors are prepared differently for their performance and are usually severely restricted from performing in terms of their own proclivities. In most cases, the theatrical actor is in a straightjacket role defined by the lines of the play.

* Bentley, *op. cit.,* pp. 185–7.

There is a parallel to this in life scenarios. Although life appears to be spontaneous, many robotlike people are as role-bound to their lives as are actors in the theater. From morning till they retire in the evening many people are restricted to specific norms and stifling rituals of behavior that parallel the demands of a rigid "life-script." Some people in their occupations (e.g., salesman, assembly line worker, etc.) are locked into a rigid role-set for behavior. The same is true for many husbands, wives, and students. In this respect, on an informal level, many people have their rigid scripts and repeat and repeat lines that they have written for themselves or that have been written for them in the process of their socialization process. They have lost their spontaneity.

This issue of being role-bound in life or an actor following a prepared theatrical script is perhaps the most significant difference between acting in theater, everyday life, and psychodrama. Psychodrama permits a greater flexibility and a larger life-space than the other forms of human expression.

In psychodrama anything is possible—incest, theft, talking to a dead person, playing one's particular God, asking for a divorce, telling off one's boss. Any act-hunger can be presented. There are few prohibitions in a psychodrama performance. The vehicle is expressly constructed for enlarging the protagonist's life-space. With the stage as a vehicle and a group of potential auxiliary egos to fill the protagonist's demands, he can enact almost any situation that his inner self demands. Psychodrama is, therefore, the only action vehicle designed exclusively for enlarging existence and deepening one's perspective on life.

In psychodrama we often utilize theatrical techniques of lighting, set, and props to aid a protagonist in presenting his story and in more coherently expressing himself. Although such theatrical elements are often used in psychodramatic sessions, psychodramatic elements have seldom been used in theatrical productions. Pirandello's *Six Characters in Search of An Author,* Genet's *The Balcony,* and Arthur Miller's *After the Fall* have psychodramatic characteristics, but other than these plays and a few others, the psychodramatic approach has not consciously been utilized in theater.

In one case, a psychodrama mood was employed in the classic film *Sunset Boulevard*. In the last scene of the film, a kind of psychodrama is produced that enabled the star of the drama, Norma Desmond, to depart into her extremist fantasies about life with grace and style. A description of the prelude to her psychodramatic departure is necessary in order to set up this poignant scene.

In the film, Norma Desmond (Gloria Swanson) is an aging superstar who has (in a psychodramatic way) maintained her stardom by blocking out the real world, which has, at this phase in her life, passed her by. She is wealthy enough, however, to perpetuate her "star status" with a doting "auxiliary ego" ex-movie director and ex-husband, Max (Erich Von Stroheim). He writes her fake fan letters and provides constant assurance of her former exalted position as a legendary Hollywood star.

She engages a young man, Joe (William Holden), to rewrite a script she has written as a vehicle for returning to her former status. For a time, he helps maintain her delusion that she will make a brilliant comeback; but then, because of his own needs—to repel her advances for a fuller relationship—he begins to introduce the realities of her age and her real position in the world.

In the climactic scene of the film, she shoots him. After killing him, the reality of her life becomes manifest to her and she retreats to another more enveloping form of isolation and pain avoidance—psychosis. In the final scene of the film, her faithful servant, ex-husband, and director, Max, sets up a regal psychodramatic scene for her arrest. Through his subtle psychodramatic direction, the police, the newsreel cameramen, and reporters all assume auxiliary ego roles. As she walks down the long staircase of her mansion toward custody, everyone in the psychodramatic cast pretends to see her as a queen leaving the real world into her deeper fantasy of stardom.

It would seem that the psychodramatic model and elements

could be employed advantageously in more theatrical productions. The use of such psychodramatic techniques as doubles, role-reversal, and soliloquy could enhance the impact of both theater and film.

All three vehicles of acting—psychodrama, theater, and life —focus on the protagonist or protagonists who are at the center of the drama. Although the leading figure or the protagonist, in psychodrama, theater, and life parallel each other in some ways, as indicated, in many respects there are some significant differences. One is that the actor in life or psychodrama can much of the time or most of the time be banal or dull. This is not true in a classic theatrical play or film.

For example, Willy Loman, the central protagonist in Arthur Miller's *Death of a Salesman,* has lines in the play that are set and brilliant. A fine actor such as Frederic March (who played Willy in the film) can enact the scenes and lines of the play and at almost every performance produce a powerful characterization that has a profound impact on an audience. This possibility does not always obtain in life. As Erich Bentley points out, many people perform inadequately in response to the expectations of life.

In addition to the constant excellence of classic theater or film, the production is always available for presentation. A theatrical team at any point in time can inflate a production for action. Partly because of this replay possibility, theater is a valuable part of the culture. Because once the drama has been artistically honed, it is always usable and uniformly effective. Every time Willy tells his two failed sons about someone—"He's liked but not well liked"— he says something of a universal nature about success in American society. In real life, Willy and his friend, Charley, could hardly rise to the power of the following brief dialogue, which provides a pungent commentary on an aspect of Willy's fantasy and the meaning of affluence and status in America:

> Charley: . . . The only thing you got in this world is what you can sell. And the funny thing is that you're a salesman, and you don't know that.

Willy: I've always tried to think otherwise, I guess. I always felt that if a man was impressive, and well liked, that nothing—
Charley: Why must everybody like you? Who liked J. P. Morgan? Was he impressive? In a Turkish bath he'd look like a butcher. But with his pockets on he was very well liked. . . .

This brilliant, sure-fire impact, which is characteristic of a classic play, does not obtain in psychodrama or in life. Although there are brilliant moments in life and psychodrama, they are different mediums of performance and do not have the *reliability* of the theater.

Despite this *reliability* advantage, the theater does lean heavily on reflecting the prototype characteristic of stereotypical characters found in the general society. The play would not have any impact if there were not hundreds of thousands of Willy Lomans in the audience or who were familiar to the audience, hungrily crying out for expression and recognition. The real-life Willy Lomans are not nearly as interesting as Miller's character, in part because before they say some clear, precise, crisp line that reveals a philosophical truth about themselves or society, they have said a thousand other things that would make most "audiences" in real life turn away from them. A brilliant playwright such as Arthur Miller is able to clip the handful of profound telling words and scenes out of the thousands actually played in life by the real-life Willy Lomans.

As portrayed by a Frederic March, Willy is never boring, whereas the Willys in real life are often painfully dull. In the play, the audience can sense the tragedy—they know how far the drama will go. In real life, Willy is a tragic figure who may unpredictably fail or drop dead at any moment. In the play, Arthur Miller beautifully and simply provides us with a character study of all the Willys. Very few of the Willys in real life would receive a poetic eulogy written by Miller and delivered at their funeral to sum up their life:

Nobody dast blame this man. You don't understand: Willy was a salesman. And for a salesman, there is no rock bottom to the life. He don't put a bolt to a nut, he don't tell you the law or give you medicine. He's a man way out there in the blue, riding on a smile and a shoeshine. And when they start not smiling back—that's an earthquake. And then you get yourself a couple of spots on your hat, and you're finished. Nobody dast blame this man. A salesman is got to dream, boy. It comes with the territory.

In Arthur Miller's superb drama, Willy has grace and style and *attention* is paid to his plight. Although psychodrama can be as uninteresting as life often is, with regard to the *attention* factor psychodrama does parallel the theater. And despite the occasional dullness of psychodrama, few sessions in which a person really bares himself in his many complexities are uninteresting.

As in a fine theatrical play, in psychodrama attention is paid. The real life "Willy" becomes the "star" of his own drama, and he is interesting because he performs the essence, the key scenes, in his life. His family and the *group* present (it is not an audience) pay close attention to his psychodramatic scenario. The director and the group provide him with every opportunity to present, examine, and reenact every significant scene in his life. In the process, he becomes bathed in the cosmetic impact of psychodrama. He becomes interesting and effusive, partly as a consequence of the group's self-interest and involvement in the session. In this regard, a psychodramatic production is like a fine play. It provides a cogent character study of the protagonist and is absorbing and fascinating to the audience-group. Psychodrama and theater are alike in that they take what is too often a dull, uninteresting life and elevate it to heroic proportions both for the protagonist and the group or audience.

In real life, friends, relatives, and sometimes strangers comprise a person's audience. In psychodrama the audience is the group present at a session. Moreno attributes a great significance to the audience—in fact, in the scheme of psychodrama, the audience is sometimes a more primary component of a session than the protagonist: "The force which releases theatre and drama is not on the stage, the actor; not behind the backdrops, the producer or the playwright; it is the audience before the proscenium. The spectator turns into an actor as he finds himself in conflict with the persons acting on the stage."

In a similar vein, Harold Clurman, in his book *On Directing,* delineates the enormous significance of the audience in theater: "Audiences differ in different places and under different conditions. It is not being 'artistic' to be unconcerned about audience reactions. To discount the nature of one's audience is to be antitheater. The audience is the theatre's prime factor and chief 'actor.' In the deepest sense it is the audience—the community or a particular segment of it—which produces the play. . . . The director chooses the spine of the play, the key or springboard of his interpretation, according to his own lights, not to mention the actors he has at his disposal, the audience he wishes to reach and the hoped-for effect on that audience, for he and his audience in a very critical sense are part of the play." *

An audience can change the entire meaning of a play. For example, the play *Arsenic and Old Lace* was directed as a thriller. On opening night, however, the audience changed it into a comedy by their reaction of uproarious laughter. The same is true of audiences in life—their response can change the meaning or the nature of an action.

"Audiences" in psychodrama, theater, and life are significantly different. In usual theater (either a live play or a movie), the audience is limited to a handful of overt responses. They can express a positive reaction through laughter, tears, or applause, boo the performance (a rare response), or, more characteristically, can remain silent. In their silence, they may be unmoved by the performance or deeply affected—yet they are limited in the scope of their reactions.

In everyday life, there is an audience that can obviously react to a protagonist. There are three basic valences of reaction: the audience or co-stars can have a positive response, a negative-re-

* Harold Clurman, *On Directing* (New York: Collier-Macmillan, 1972), p. 20.

jecting response, or can be indifferent without any concrete reaction.

In psychodrama there is direction, and "the audience" can and often does get right on the stage and into the protagonist's life. They may—if it's appropriate—double with the protagonist, or a member of the group may play a son or wife. The audience may and often does experience the protagonist's pain, joy, catharsis, and insights. They learn from the protagonist and teach him from their own experience. Unlike the staged drama, in which everything is preset and the audience is barricaded from the stage and to a great extent from enacting their emotions, in psychodrama almost everything goes, except any action that will hurt the protagonist. The "audience" in psychodrama, therefore, is symbolically and actually merged with the protagonist in his drama.

Everyone performs a variety of roles in life. Most of the time, the varied roles are enacted on different sets and there is limited confusion about the actor's performance. Sometimes, however, an actor encounters the confusion of role conflict. This emerges when the actor is confronted at the same moment with two divergent and conflicting sets of expectation in a situation. For example, a young man plays a childlike "momma's boy" when he is with his mother and a man of the world with his wife. When he finds himself in the company of both his wife and mother on the same life set, he may manifest a form of role conflict or role confusion. The wife expects him to act like a "man," an adult; the mother expects him to act like her little boy and to conform to her every command.

Theatrical actors sometimes have a special problem of role conflict when they play roles alien to the way they are in terms of their own self or basic personality. The theatrical process of being or becoming someone else often affects their personal life or their theatrical performance. This problem may be termed the *histrionic symdrome:* the condition in which a threatrical actor confuses his personal identity with his role. The histrionic syndrome is a complex problem of identity and role confusion that has meaning not only for theatrical actors but for acting in everyday life because of the element of role conflict.

Moreno describes an aspect of this phenomenon as the histrionic neurosis: "the actor has to identify himself with hundreds of roles in the course of his professional life which are alien to his own psyche. Often he has to prostitute his private psyche, to push it aside and ruin it. A split develops between his private life as father, husband, lover, businessman and the repertory of corresponding roles he has to play in the theater—a kind of 'histrionic neurosis.' Histrionic neurosis is to the actor what flat feet are to the waiter, an occupational hazard."

In the following analysis of the issue of the *histrionic syndrome* as it relates to acting in everyday life, psychodrama, and the theater, I will use the case of George Raft, the movie star of the thirties. (I have two simple reasons for using Raft as the center of this discussion: (1) his film career exemplifies the meaning of the histrionic syndrome; and (2) I spent three years studying Raft's life with an emphasis on this issue in the process of writing his biography, *George Raft,* McGraw-Hill, 1974.)

In the process of writing Raft's biography, I spent over a hundred hours in personal discussion with the actor and found Raft to be a man who had a profound problem most of his life with the histrionic syndrome.

When Raft worked at Warner Brothers in the thirties and forties, he became part of a star system that included many fine actors such as Edward G. Robinson, Bette Davis, Paul Muni, and James Cagney. For these actors, unlike Raft, there was usually a limited confusion between the roles they played and their personal identity. George Raft, however, invariably played himself on the screen, and this fostered his histrionic syndrome. In brief, the other actors used an acting skill to portray a role, whereas Raft tended to portray a character based to a great extent on roles he had actually played in life. Raft's personal relationship to his theatrical roles was complex.

Raft's cool screen facade masked a man plagued by phobias, nervous habits, and hidden fears. His feelings about himself were sometimes so negative that he looked into a mirror only when he combed his hair, and then he rushed the process. Since his earliest movies, Raft consistently refused to view himself on the screen. After he saw his first movies, he refused to see the rushes, rough cuts, or even the final prints of any of his subsequent films. Once, in an appearance on the Johnny Carson talk show, Carson showed an old film clip of Raft's movie *Bolero* and was amazed to see Raft turn away. When Carson questioned him, Raft replied, "I'm afraid to look, because I'm probably awful." The other actors cited, did not see their "self," when they looked at themselves on the screen; they saw a performance. But Raft's involvement with the roles he played and his low self-concept made it painful for him to see *his* actual "self" on the screen.

In real life, Raft had battled his way to stardom from a childhood of poverty in Hell's Kitchen, New York. In Raft's later years, when he became an affluent Hollywood film star, he was like the "Golden Boy" of Clifford Odets' great play. In a commentary on this play, about a fighter who rose up from poverty, Harold Clurman made a penetrating comment on what might be called The Golden Boy Syndrome. It characterizes George Raft's life and is revealing about what later led to his personal problems of role confusion on and off the screen.

> The story of this play is not so much the story of a prize-fighter as the picture of a great fight—a fight in which we are all involved, whatever our profession or craft. What the golden boy of this allegory is fighting for is a place in the world as an individual; what he wants is to free his ego from the scorn that attaches to "nobodies" in a society in which every activity is viewed in the light of a competition. He wants success not simply for the soft life—automobiles, etc.—which he talks about, but because the acclaim that goes with it promises him acceptance by the world, peace with it, safety from becoming the victim that it makes of the poor, the alien, the unnoticed minorities. To achieve this success, he must exploit an accidental attribute of his make-up, a mere skill, and abandon the development of his real self.*

* Harold Clurman in Clifford Odets, *Six Plays of Clifford Odets* (New York: Random House, 1939), p. 430.

In Raft's case, the attribute was his tough-guy looks, his style, and his flip-of-the-coin gambler attitude on the screen. This he had acquired from being a dancer on Broadway, hanging out with real-life gangsters, and being a part-time hood himself, involved wtih bootlegging during Prohibition.

In a peculiar way, Raft believed that the roles he was asked to play represented his personal self. He once told me, "I was offered this part of a judge who is so corrupt he pushes dope. *I could never do that!*" In this way, he tended to personalize the characters he was called upon to play and more than once refused to play purely evil roles. When he did agree to play ruthless, wholly evil characters on the screen, he insisted on being killed at the end of the film. He also felt there were some portraitures that were too unsavory or repellent for him to play, under any circumstances. One such rejection of a role led to the first of his many suspensions from Paramount—all for similar reasons.

An example of his stance on this issue and his role confusion as a gangster or a good guy is revealed by a role he rejected in the early 1930s in a film that had the working title *The Shame of Temple Drake*. The film involved a psychopathic character, Popeye, who raped a girl with a corncob and then killed her feeble-minded son. The film was based on William Faulkner's book *Sanctuary,* and, in the context of the studio system of the 1930s, the Popeye role was assigned by Paramount to Raft.

In the novel by Faulkner, the character Popeye was described in several scattered passages as: "A man of under size, a cigarette slanted from his chin. His face has a queer bloodless color as though seen by electric light; in his slanted straw hat and slightly akimbo arms he had the vicious depthless quality of stamped tin. . . . He twisted and pinched cigarettes in his little doll-like hands. His skin had a dead dark pallor. He had no chin at all. His face just went away like the face of a wax doll set too near a hot fire. . . . Popeye's eyes looked like rubber knobs. . . . Popeye looked about with a sort of vicious cringing."

As if Popeye's appearance wasn't horrendous enough, he also, according to the story, either had no penis (an unthinkable condition for swordsman George Raft) or had been castrated for a crime committed in another town. In one passage in *Sanctuary*, a doctor says, "He will never be a man, properly speaking."

Raft absolutely refused to play the role, even though his suspension by the studio cost him a considerable amount of money. His peculiar histrionic syndrome and role confusion became manifest in one of his diatribes at that time about "being" Popeye: "That part was plain suicide for me—a fellow with my face. Any other actor might play it and maybe get away with it, but I *look like that kind of a guy*. Not just on the screen—on the street, anywhere. There'd be just one thing for the public to think—'George Raft is Popeye.' "

George's personal and screen role conflict manifested itself in another parallel situation. He was asked by film mogul Samuel Goldwyn to play the part of Baby Face Martin in the film called *Dead End*. In the role, he was to become a psychopathic killer sought by the police who hides out in the New York slum where he was raised as a boy. Raft balked at one particular facet of Martin's character: "Here I am, on the lam, hiding out around this neighborhood in cellars and places like that and I meet this gang of kids. One gang member recognizes me as this killer, Baby Face Martin. The gang begins to idolize me—and I'm supposed to teach these kids how to be tough and how to be a criminal. I couldn't bring myself to do that.

"I told Mr. Goldwyn how I would like to play the part. I want a scene where I tell the kids how bad my life is, 'Just look at me crawling around like a rat, hiding. You don't want to hide all your life. Make something of yourself. Don't grow up like me.'

"In another scene I'm supposed to be with my mother and she slaps my face and calls me 'a no-good bum.' The way they had it I was just supposed to walk away mad. I wanted to play it with a tear in my eye, so the audience knows that my mother is right, and that I feel bad about my life as a criminal."

Raft's insistence at not playing these roles reveals his histrionic syndrome. He tended to confuse his *own self* with the theatrical roles he was asked to perform for film.

This type of histrionic syndrome problem emerges when an actor's self-identity becomes schizoid. A role conflict about who the person really is becomes confused with his theatrical identity. As an actor's wife who had the problem once told me, "When my husband comes home, I don't know whether it's going to be my husband Joe, King Lear, or John Dillinger."

Some facets of this syndrome are cogently portrayed in the film *A Double Life* (1944). Ronald Coleman, in the movie, portrays a Shakespearean actor embroiled in the role of Othello. After performing the intense act of killing Desdemona on stage every night for over a year, the actor's personal life became complicated by the role he played in the drama. He becomes driven to exorcise the now demon role of Othello that begins to take over his life. He meets a blonde waitress (played by Shelley Winters) who becomes his off-screen Desdemona and with whom he has an affair. In the film, she becomes frightened as his conversations with her lapse into the explicit hysterical, jealous, and accusatory speeches of Shakespeare's Othello. The theatrical role finally dominates his personal identity, and the actor in the film actually kills the waitress, his "real life" Desdemona.

The histrionic syndrome involves an overlap between the roles the actor *plays* in theater and his personal identity. The average person may have identity problems, but he usually knows who he is better than many actors. John Smith plays John Smith, and he does not usually have the *acting instrument* to play Hamlet or any other role foreign to his personal life. As a result of his training, an actor can slip rapidly into a role that is not himself. If an actor is not super-careful about his trained facility to take on a foreign extra-self role, his personal identity may become drowned by the acting roles he plays professionally. If, as in the case of "Raft as gangster," the role is persistent and consistent, the individual's personal identity becomes submerged by the parts he plays, or else he fears this will happen.

Because of these complex conditions, professional actors are not usually good protagonists in psychodrama. They often manifest a degree of confusion between their role in life and the roles they have played in the theater. Also, unlike most people, they have developed a *technique for playing parts foreign to their real selves*. Often in psychodrama, they slip into a part (either as a protagonist or auxiliary ego) and this shields them from confronting a situation as their *self*. People who are not in the theater do not usually have this facility—and consequently are forced to *be* as they are in reality. The most effective role the average person can play (even when he is not satisfied with the part) is *his own*, and this is the role that is a requisite to good psychodrama.

A SUMMARY OF COMMON ELEMENTS OF PERFORMANCE

There are many additional commentaries that can be made about the parallels and differences between psychodrama, theater, and life. In summary, I would note that although there is considerable overlap, role performances in these three basic genres of human behavior have distinctly different requirements. These can be best delineated by examining people's performance in terms of some common elements.

The theater, everyday life, and psychodrama have several specific elements in common that further help to delineate their relationships. These include motivation, the set, the cast, the audience, and the scenario.

Motivation. There is an act-hunger that motivates people in everyday life. The motivations are varied. They exist, among other reasons, for the satisfaction of physiological and psychological needs.

In the theater, motivation involves the actor examining the motivation of the external (at least to his self) character he is to play in the overall drama. It requires an analysis of what drives the person in the total drama of that character—and how he would perform in the specific scenes being played.

The motivation in psychodrama relates to the protagonist's problem in real life. He is motivated to play scenes to cathart and to comprehend certain phenomena in his life. The stage actor is concerned primarily with the goal of a good performance in a play that will have impact on a theatrical audience; the protagonist's goal in psychodrama is to resolve a personal dilemma or problem that will make him a more effective performer in life.

The Set. In everyday life, people perform on various types of sets. Their home, or basic living quarters, is usually their essential *set*. A person's set in everyday life is not always within the frame of his control. For example, someone who is relatively poor may dream of a luxurious set that is beyond his financial grasp.

In the theater, a set may be opulent or stark. Some sets are purposefully bare in order to focus the actors more intensively. In psychodrama the set is constructed according to the protagonist's mind's eye in a given situation and is very revealing about the performer. The protagonist is asked to set up the scene, usually with just a few simple chairs and a table. The protagonist will soliloquize the colors and the opulence (or lack of it) of the set on which he is to perform an emotional scene. This set has considerable meaning for his emotional mood. In psychodrama some people go into a great and meticulous description of their set. For others, who are not as involved with this facet of their life, the construction of their set in a session is quick and modest. Whatever a protagonist does is revealing. For example, I recall one very compulsive protagonist who meticulously set up a table with two chairs in his kitchen, where he was to play an emotional scene. To test my hypothesis about his compulsiveness, when he wasn't looking I moved the table about six inches from the spot where he had placed it. Several minutes later, when he noticed that the table was not on the mark he set, he felt compelled to move the table back to its *exact* original position. This act revealed and confirmed something emotionally meaningful about the protagonist's compulsive nature that later emerged more concretely in the session.

The Cast. In psychodrama there are no fixed co-stars or cast. In most scenes, the protagonist can select his own auxiliary ego cast and through role reversal set them up to perform in any way he desires. In life people drop or replace their co-stars through moving, divorce, or changing employment. Psychodrama provides the opportunity to "screen-test" or role-test potential co-stars for a person's life cast.

The *cast* in a psychodrama is usually comprised of auxiliary egos from the group. There are three ways to cast an auxiliary ego for a scene in a psychodrama: (1) The protagonist may select the person in the group he feels will best play the required role (e.g., mother, father, spouse, child) because of the way that person looks or the emotional vibrations he feels from the person; (2) the director may "cast the part" with someone he (a) believes will give an effective emotional portrayal for the benefit of the protagonist, or (b) because he believes the enactment of the particular auxiliary ego role will be emotionally beneficial *to the auxiliary ego* as well as to the protagonist; and (3) a member of the group may be emotionally warmed up to play the role and volunteer for the part.

Casting in psychodrama is a delicate, complex, and highly significant action. For example, in working on the casting issue for a television program on psychodrama, it was suggested that a repertory team of theatrical actors should be available to me as auxiliary egos. It was further determined for semantic reasons to call such auxiliary egos "psychodramatic actors."

The problem I found with most exclusively trained-for-theatrical-performance actors in psychodrama is that they are geared essentially to a "larger-than-life" performance (that has "production value") for maximum impact on an audience. In classic psychodrama, an auxiliary ego cast for a role has as his *first priority* the humanistic-emotional obligation to fulfill the protagonist's image of the auxiliary role as an extension of the protagonist so that the protagonist can objectify, explicate, and explore his inner monodrama. A second and most important responsibility of a psychodramatic auxiliary ego is to function as a therapeutic extension of the psychodrama director for the purpose of insuring maximum therapeutic intervention.

Often the performance of a trained theatrical actor, no matter how great an actor he or she may be, is an assault on the emotional integrity and requirements of the protagonist and the session because the psychodrama actor tends to play a role for his own ego needs of a "good performance" for an audience. This is not always the case because, of course, some rare actors, trained in both theater and psychodrama, can by their performance fulfill both requirements—their ethical and emotional obligations to the protagonist and his problem, and a broad acting skill that has a profound impact on an audience. This type of ideal enactment also requires the subtle attribute of *not* upstaging the protagonist.

In regard to casting theatrical actors for a psychodramatic mass audience vehicle, there are at least two possible effects, neither of which has been clearly proven. One assumption is that an actor is trained to have an emotional impact on an audience, and in the mass media it is advantageous to have a "larger-than-life" performance in order to achieve maximum impact. The other position I am inclined to favor is that a psychodramatic production focusing *on the protagonist* by casting psychologically oriented, sensitive auxiliary egos (who are not acting in the theatrical sense) in the psychodrama will have the greatest emotional impact and the most significant personal meaning to the largest audience; and I would add that this type of program would also have the greatest entertainment value for a mass audience. The result would be my ideal desired goal of producing a uniquely entertaining production for a mass audience that will also have a beneficial therapeutic impact.

There is, of course, no blockade to utilizing an ideal cast for mass-media psychodrama that would combine a repertory group of both psychodramatically oriented theatrical actors and theatrically oriented trained auxiliary egos. Both types of profesionals would comprise an effective cast for a mass theatrical psychodrama.

A central issue in psychodrama—as in life—is how specific and particular a protagonist can be in selecting a cast for his personal production. How many times have people been amazed at someone's selection of a husband or wife? The "casting" of a spouse in real life may be totally out of the consensual definition of the person's circle of friends and acquaintances. In a parallel way, in psychodrama protagonists tend to be most precise about their casting.

As one example, I recall a session in which Moreno was casting the role of the Devil to fulfill the requirements of a scene for a hospitalized patient's fantasy. After attempting to cast about ten people from the group—all of whom were considered wrong for the part by the protagonist—Moreno brought me on stage as the lady's Satan. Before I could utter a word or present any emotional expression, her face beamed with approval, and she pointed at me and announced to the world, "That is the Devil!!" Warmed up by proper casting, she launched into one of the most poignant, profound, and dramatic psychodramas I had ever participated in, one that drew everyone in the group into her exotic fantasy world. The process had the ultimate effect of producing trust in a person who had been so alienated that she had rejected the consensual reality of the world most people inhabit. The proper casting of her devil became *the key* to her acceptance of the group present and eventually to more people and groups in society. An analagous process often happens in the real world for people less emotionally disturbed or isolated when they successfully "cast" a significant person into their life.

The Audience. There is usually an audience in everyday life. Even when a person is alone, he is often involved with his audience. A person dressing before a mirror is not looking at himself alone but is anticipating his audience. A person morosely alone may be angered because he anticipates his audience will not approve of him. *Paranoia provides an audience.* In fact, in a group, *all others* are the audience to what one says or does. The audience may be harsh or approving, depending on the appropriateness of a person's action in everyday life.

Most people in everyday life have an audience of only one or two people who count. Others, such as theatrical stars, envision and sometimes emotionally require an audience or a cast of thousands.

In the theater, the audience is generally immobile. They can display their reaction only in several forms: applause, laughter, tears, walking out, or staying away from the performance. Writer-critics are the kings and queens of an audience to a theatrical actor. Some actors or stars, like most people, revere their audiences; others have disdain.

In psychodrama the audience is a function of the protagonist. The audience is not there in a spectator's role but is there to support, to co-exist, to act in concert with the protagonist. The audience group is present to help the subject of the session construct his required drama and analyze and understand his life behavior. They are expected primarily to be compassionate, sympathetic co-actors. They assume a critical or analytic role at the end of the protagonist's performance when they share their own experiences.

The Scenario or Script. In everyday life, most people *do not act but react* to their drama as it is dictated by others rather than being in full control of their scenario or script. Often, in robotlike fashion, they conform to a cultural script that seems to be, or that they accept to be, their fate. In this regard, they are role-bound to try to achieve or replicate a frozen script.

One lady revealed in psychodrama that in her *life struggle* or scenario she has a "Little Orphan Annie-Daddy Warbucks" script that has controlled her life. She is always the little waif looking for this strong, rich, older man to take over and provide her with an entertaining life of affluence. She seldom found the co-star that would help her to enact the scenario on which she had fixated, and she spent most of her days depressed and pining away for a desired affluent co-star who never appeared except in her fantasy.

In another, more complex, role-bound script, Alicia, a young lady of about twenty, presented a psychodrama in which her guiding life struggle was an attempt to be accepted as an adult by her mother and father. In several "acts," she presented scenes in which she tried to crack into the tight dyad of her mother-father. In the last act of her session, Alicia presented a complex set of maneuvers through which the boyfriend she "loved" wound up as the boyfriend and lover of her "best friend"—partly through Alicia's own subtle manipulation. As she was enacting her current painful effort to now crack through the become part of her boyfriend-girlfriend dyad, perceptive members of the group present at the session pointed out to her in the post-discussion how she had replicated the basic life struggle she had with her parents. This pattern of replicating an early life struggle is a generic construct I often find in the life script of many psychodramatic protagonists. Scenarios are obviously even more highly structured in theater than in psychodrama, except in psychodrama there is a much greater possibility for revising the script. In theater this is not possible except in some rare productions that permit a degree of acting spontaneity and creativity. In theater the role of Hamlet may have some dimensions for interpretation, but for the most part the dialogue and drama is set. There is no happy ending in sight for Hamlet without dramatically altering the fixed script.

In psychodrama there is almost complete freedom for a protagonist to "write" his own drama. In fact, this is a central attribute of psychodrama. The protagonist has almost complete freedom to break out of the script composed for him in his early years and by everyday life—to produce his own drama, dialogue, and script *on his own terms*. Part of the fulfillment of psychodrama is to write one's own script, to write and act out one's own conclusion, to leave the beaten path and explore the emotions of a new life direction.

This facet of psychodrama that is different from everyday life and the confines of a theatrical performance is the acting-out of a "surplus-reality." Behavior may be exaggerated to almost caricature dimensions for the purpose of understanding and experience. For example, a father, the protagonist in a session, in a scene scolded his son for his misbehavior. The auxiliary ego playing the role of the man's son reversed roles with the father. The real father became the son. The auxiliary ego as the father began to shout and manhandle the "son" (the real father), who cowered in stark terror at the blast of surplus-reality. When the role-playing stopped, the father admitted that in the role of the son he was terrorized. But he then quickly remarked, "Of course this was exaggerated. I never yell that loud or push my son that hard." The group and the director reminded him that that was his version, and that the son, from his point of view, might be experiencing a snarling ogre of a father. Thus, the surplus-reality of psychodrama can often get a message through to someone more intensively than simply talking to the person about the situation. The same extremist performance in everyday life could have deleterious effects and, if done in the theater, might not be believed, because it did not seem "true-to-life."

Another characteristic of psychodrama, compared to the theater, is the *flexibility* factor of a scenario. A protagonist can play the entire cast of his social atom; that is, a man, in a session, through the technique of role reversal, may play his son, his wife, his mother, his employer, his minister, etc. From these other role vantage points, he can see other dimensions of himself.

Also, as indicated, psychodrama is not *time-bound* like life and, in most respects, the theater. A scenario can have a past, present, or future reference point. In everyday life, we can remember life in the moment or project ourselves into the future, but if we move out of the present, it doesn't have the definitiveness of a psychodrama situation. In the theater, the actors are even more definitely locked into the time situation set by the playwright in a script that is preset.

In all of these contexts, we should not view psychodrama *exclusively* as a vehicle for possible *social change* or *therapy;* it is also a human behavior pattern that enables a person to live out a fuller, wider life pattern.

As in Genet's *The Balcony,* in which illusions were created for enacting a broader sexual fantasy, or as in *Six Characters in*

Search of an Author, in which the characters were looking for a life stage on which to act-out their problems, in psychodrama there is the possibility (therapy aside) for telling your boss off, telling your spouse what you really think of him or her, or doing a life-swap (becoming a millionaire or a star of your choice). All of these desired roles can be played out in psychodrama without the protagonist being viewed as psychotic, penalized, or locked up for law violation. Although the experience may not be precisely what the role-occupant would experience in that role in everyday life, the "surplus-reality" of psychodrama does provide the opportunity for experiencing a broader range of life roles and situations than the person confronts in everyday life or in the theater.

To achieve complete and full *stardom* in his own production, the protagonist has the right to select any co-stars (auxiliary egos) he desires; to perform any scenes of fantasy and/or imagination; and to eliminate time boundaries by going back to childhood, forward to the cosmic future, or even into psychosis or death.

Of the three generic forms of human interaction, psychodrama provides the greatest freedom and potential, at least in the here-and-now of the session. It enables a person to explore and explicate with a totally cooperative audience and director the many directions of the scenarios that exist in the monodrama of his psyche. The psychodramatic process of human behavior may thus help a person to successfully revise and emotionally experience significant scenarios of his everyday life in a creative and productive new way—a way that can enlarge his perspective and existence.

CHAPTER

7

Psychodrama in Society

I N HIS now classic book, *Who Shall Survive?* Moreno makes a seemingly megalomaniacal statement: "A truly therapeutic method can not have less a goal than the totality of mankind." *

An assumption of this psychodramatic concept is that all people in society are related in some fashion and that when any person is changed in any way it alters that person and his network of relationships. It also implies that "the group" or the "social atom" is the fundamental unit of society rather than the individual; and that any social change taking place in small groups affects the larger society.

Moving from the framework of the general society to a particular social institution, such as the family, it is apparent that when any member of a family has his personality modified it

* J. L. Moreno, *Who Shall Survive?* (New York: Beacon House, 1953), p. 3.

alters the relationships of the entire family. In reverse, in this same context of logic, if a member of a family is pathological, the roots of the problem can be found in the family's social structure. The child may become the family "scapegoat" and, thus, the symptomatic carrier of a family pathology that stems not necessarily from the youth's personality or personal motivation but from the family's particular structure.

In this regard, psychologist Eric Bermann, in his book *Scapegoat*, describes how an eight-year-old boy's personal problems and subsequent delinquent behavior resulted from an effort to repress the family's general problem.*

In his work with the family, Dr. Bermann learned that the father attempted to conceal the fact that he had a heart condition, was in need of open-heart surgery, and was medically considered "close to death" for many years. The family repressed their awareness of the condition and seldom openly talked about the sword of doom that hung over their lives. The problem, Dr. Bermann noted, created terrible tensions that were acted out obliquely on the one son, Roscoe, during his early years. According to Bermann, "with each succeeding visit I began to understand further the depth of the family's trouble. Their terror and desperation of the 'tactics' for avoiding overt recognition of an ever present death-fear became apparent. . . . It became increasingly clear that in the face of their overwhelming dread, this family of seven had—in collusive but entirely nonconscious and unspoken fashion —selected Roscoe as their scapegoat."

In this subtle way, the family colluded to make Roscoe the problem. They seldom talked to him or acknowledged his presence. His spirit was broken at home. He conformed when he was at home, but on the outside he began to act out his hostility in delinquent ways. According to Bermann: "Once trained and fit into the scapegoat role, the child becomes indispensable to his family. He provided a center for their grievances in a highly

* Eric Bermann, *Scapegoat* (Ann Arbor: University of Michigan Press, 1973).

efficient and automatic fashion, and, as whipping boy, stabilized the social system of the family."

Roscoe's delinquent behavior began at the age of eight, stemming from his father's problem and the family reaction, and continued into his teenage years. He was viewed by society and its helping agencies as a child with a personal problem. In fact, his behavior was a function of the family's structural problems, which stemmed from his father's physical disability. As the "scapegoat," he was arrested over five times, and his delinquent career was fostered by the further negative socialization of deviance in juvenile detention. It is important to understand a person's family and its sociometric structure in order to understand his or her pathological behavior.

Based on this fundamental concept, it is axiomatic in all psychodrama sessions with one member of a family to keep the entire sociometric structure of the family in mind as a blueprint for the family group's therapy. *In this same context in psychodrama, an effective director is always aware that the modification of any individual's role in a group invariably affects the larger society.*

Related to this psychodramatic principle, I vividly recall another case of a sociometric problem in a family that produced a severe pathology in one member of the family. Herbie, age eleven, came to Moreno's Beacon Sanitorium after spending a brief period at a state hospital, where he was diagnosed as psychotic. His parents, who were affluent, felt guilty about keeping him in a state hospital, heard about Moreno's sanitorium, and brought him there for treatment.

I worked with Dr. Moreno in several sessions he directed with this frail, super-sensitive youngster. Herbie was almost in a catatonic state of withdrawal during his first session. I played the role of his father in several sessions. Herbie began to open up and finally expressed his enormous hostility toward his mother and father. The most productive information was revealed in devastating cameo statements when he reversed roles and assumed the role of his father when he was drunk (a common occurrence).

The manner in which Herbie was typecast in the "sick" role is indicated by his alcoholic father's harangues.

HERBIE AS HIS FATHER: You little bastard, I never wanted you in the first place. If you weren't such a goddamn problem, I would quit drinking. *You made me an alcoholic!* Because of *you* I can't even hold a job. You've ruined our family.

Herbie's mother was also a significant negative force in driving him out of this world of painful reality into a withdrawn dream-world where he was cast as a psychotic.

HERBIE AS MOTHER: I love you, my sweet boy. I feel awful about what's happening to you. But really if it weren't for you I'd still have my husband. After you were born everything went wrong. It's not your fault—but you were a mistake. Your dad wasn't ready to be a father.

In this triad (there were no other children), the parents projected their problems onto Herbie, in an effort to rationalize their own deficiencies. The parents unconsciously had a vested interest in keeping Herbie in the "sick" role despite overt protestations to the contrary. If Herbie was "sick," they could rationalize their own stigmatized problems by blaming *him* for their troubles. Herbie's reaction to this unbearable pressure at eleven was to retreat from the painful world of his family's reality into a cocoon of fantasy. He almost had to do this in order to survive. In order to understand Herbie's personality problem, it was vital to understand the sociometry of his family—and to some extent the society in which the seemingly individual problem had emerged.

In a variety of psychodrama sessions with his parents that included discussions of Herbie's social atom and his family, Herbie's problems were somewhat relieved. When the pressure was taken off Herbie through placement in a reasonable foster family setting, he made considerable progress in the resolution of his problem. Without Herbie to blame, the parents had to seek help for their problems. And without this mother and father, other more constructive role possibilities opened up for Herbie. *It is, therefore, vital to understand the social atom of an individual, the roles he is cast in, and the sociometry of the family in society to utilize psychodrama properly.*

In psychodrama the social atom, not the individual, is considered the smallest social unit. The social atom refers to an individual *and* the configuration of people (near or distant) to whom he is emotionally related. Sociometric research reveals that the constellation of a social atom functions as a unit.

A person's social atom changes from time to time in membership, but there is a consistency about its structure. An individual has from birth a structure of relationships around him; mother, father, brothers, or sisters. As he grows older, he enlarges the size of his social atom. A person who is effective in life develops a system of relationships that is vibrant and satisfying.

Moreno contends that beyond a certain age, for most people, it becomes increasingly difficult to replace lost relationships and "social death" begins to parallel physiological death.* Social death becomes significant to most people before physical or mental death. An individual's social atom deteriorates for various reasons: (a) the loss of the affection of a loved one, (b) the replacement of an individual in a person's configuration by someone who is not as adequate, and (c) death. The death of a crucial person in a person's social atom is often shocking and highly significant to the survivor. In this respect, we die in small and large ways, depending upon the strength of our relationships. "Getting old" in Western societies is generally considered a terrible state of being, and "old people" in our society tend to give in to their continuing situation of social deaths. People can withstand these impacts and should restore their losses with new friends, since people feel death as their social atom dies. Through the psychodramatic encouragement of love and spontaneity, people can maintain their youthful attractiveness beyond the boundaries of age that are stereotyped by societal norms.

* J. L. Moreno, "The Social Atom and Death" in *Sociometry, Experimental Method, and The Science of Society* (New York: Beacon House, 1951), p. 65.

Psychodrama is a part of a triad of approaches that includes *sociometry* and *sociodrama*. In this conceptual scheme, sociometry is the method for ascertaining a group's structure by having the participants reveal their emotional attractions, rejections, and neutrality toward each other in the small groups that comprise the larger social system; *sociodrama* is a method of role-playing in a group to explore interior emotions about certain social constellations, such as racism, parent-child interaction, or husband-wife conflict; and *psychodrama* of course, is the method of role-playing that uses a system of devices for getting people to live together more spontaneously, creatively, and with greater compassion and enhances the ability of a person to perform more effectively in life.

Psychodrama is the master action system that encompasses sociometry and sociodrama, and it is the fountainhead of many recent innovative group approaches. It contains diagnostic procedures as well as emotion-affecting strategies. At the center of the theory of psychodrama are the concepts of *spontaneity, creativity,* and the *cultural conserves* of human behavior.

In order for *creativity* in human behavior to come alive, there must be spontaneity. According to Moreno, "Creativity is a sleeping beauty that, in order to become effective, needs a catalyzer. The arch catalyzer of creativity is spontaneity." Spontaneity is an essential characteristic of psychodrama. It involves learning the ability to respond adequately and effectively in human interaction. Spontaneity training develops the ability in an individual to respond *adequately to a new situation or to enact a new response to an old situation.* The overall aim of "spontaneity training" in psychodrama is to develop more creative, effective, self-fulfilled role-playing in life.

Another result of increased spontaneity and creativity in social interaction is the *cultural conserve.* Moreno states, "The finished product of the creative process is the *cultural conserve,* which comes from *conservare.* It is anything that preserves the value of a particular culture." A *conserve* may take the form of a material object, such as a book, film, or building, or it may appear as a highly set pattern of behavior, such as a ceremony, a ritual, a language, or a concept. The *conserve* is important, since without it people would have to recreate the same cultural forms daily to meet life situations.

In addition to providing continuity to the perpetuation of human existence, the cultural conserve plays an even more significant role as a springboard for catalyzing new spontaneity and creativity. For example, reading a conserve—such as a book—or seeing an exciting film may inspire great creativity. The conserve, therefore, has its own value, if utilized properly in people's lives, in fostering creativity.

The established culture, and its folkways and mores, is of great value in society; however, there is a danger in over-reliance on the conserve. If people do not utilize and exercise their human spontaneity and creativity in life or develop it in psychodrama, they may become over-reliant on the crutches of conserves and run the risk of becoming robotlike in their behavior. This risk factor seems to be greatest in contemporary technocratic societies.

Super-technocratic societies have a special problem with the machine enslavement of people. People are in constant conflict with the machines of their creation and run the risk of being dominated by the machinelike Golems they produce. Technocratic developments have always had two edges: one that benefits people and another dimension that is potentially destructive. Prior to this century, however, technology and human survival was not the critical issue it is today.

Among Moreno's many pertinent observations on people and machines in *Who Shall Survive?* was the haunting speculation: "The fate of man threatens to become that of the dinosaur in reverse. The dinosaur may have perished because he extended the power of his organism in excess of its usefulness. Man may perish because of reducing the power of his organism by fabricating robots [machines] in excess of his control." *

Paradoxically, although it is increasingly a distinct possibility,

* Moreno, "The Social Atom and Death," p. 604.

the final outcome of people versus their technological robots may not be the total physical annihilation of people. People may in a subtle fashion become robotlike in their interaction and become human robots. This more insidious conclusion to the present course of action would be the silent disappearance of *human* interaction. In another kind of death, *social death,* people would be oppressively locked into robotlike roles in groups that had become *social machines.* In this context, social death at various chronological ages would appear in the form of people mouthing ahuman, regimented platitudes—playing a robot role—on a meaningless, dead stage of everyday life.

The essence of the problem is that if people become subservient to the machines they produce, they would lose their basic vital creative ability. In Moreno's terms, people would tend to become "technocrats" rather than "creatocrats." Technocrats are people more dependent on their machines than creatocrats, who are people concerned with developing their creative abilities for the purpose of becoming more humanistic in their social relationships.

The submission of people to their machines is a subtle process. It seems that the more machines people produce, the more their creative abilities and resources are diminished. People would ultimately become dependent on the precise and effective machines they had produced and lose their fundamental humanistic-creative ability.

Part of the reason for people's preoccupation with creating machines (cultural conserves), is their fear of the unknown. They fear the exigencies of the future and attempt to store up power and patterns of behavior for expected and imminent crises. They do not trust their own spontaneity and creativity, so they package it in a machine, or a *cultural conserve.* Machines have better memories than people and, in some cases, function more efficiently; consequently, more and more people become more and more dependent on machines. Moreno warns that people in this process can ultimately lose their spontaneity and creative ability—

the *primary* characteristic of being human: "As our perfectionism has failed us again and again in its application to us as biological and social beings, as individuals and as a society of individuals, we give up hope and invest it in zoomatons [robots]. The pathological consequences are enormous. Man turns more and more into a function of cultural and technological conserves, puts a premium on power and efficiency and loses credence in spontaneity and creativity." *

In my book *Robopaths: People as Machines,* I attempt to examine contemporary Western social systems in the context of Moreno's fundamental theories of human society.† In the process, I coined the word *robopath* to describe people who have suffered the affliction of social death in their lives to the point where they enact robot roles. Although psychodrama is a method for dealing with a variety of human dilemmas and problems, it was conceived by Moreno in its most significant sense as a vehicle for counterattacking the growing problem of robopathology in individuals and the larger problem of the death of a humanistic society.

The term *robopath* (meaning the pathology of robot behavior) has its roots in the word *robot,* introduced into the language in 1923 by the Czechoslovakian writer Karel Čapek in a play title *R. U. R.* The letters stand for Rossum's Universal Robots, the centerpiece of a classic science fiction play about a factory that manufactured humanlike machine robots for worldwide use.

The formula for the robots was created by an inventor named Rossum. Early in the play, Rossum's son, head of the plant since his father's death, comments about his father:

> He invented a worker with the minimum amount of requirements. He had to simplify him. He rejected everything that did not contribute directly to the progress of work. In this way he rejected man and made the Robot. Robots are not people. Me-

* Moreno, "The Social Atom and Death," p. 604.
† Parts of this segment are derived from my book, *Robopaths: People as Machines* (New York: Bobbs-Merrill, 1972, Penguin Books, 1973).

chanically they are more perfect than we are, they have an enormously developed intelligence, but they have no soul. . . .

They've astonishing memories, you know. If you were to read a twenty-volume Encyclopaedia to them, they'd repeat it all to you with absolute accuracy. But they never think of anything new.*

In the story line of the play, the robots rebel against their human masters, organize, and begin to assume power by systematically killing off the people who created them. Toward the end of *R.U.R.*, the robot leaders plead for help from a scientist who is the only human left in the world. They desperately need his help with their central dilemma, the problem of reproducing themselves. If they do not learn the formula for reproduction from this scientist, they will become extinct.

The contemporary problems of the automation of people, megamachines, and potential ecological and social death have some interesting parallels with Čapek's remarkable literary predictions. In the play, Dr. Gall, the director of the robot plant, responds to an inquisitive woman's questions about the potential of self-destruction by the rising growth of robots. His response, interestingly, parallels the commentary of many bureaucrats and politicians on the contemporary scene.

> Dr. Gall: Because the Robots are being manufactured, there's a surplus of labour supplies. So people are becoming superfluous, unnecessary so to speak. Man is really a survivor. But that he should begin to die out after a paltry thirty years of competition—that's the awful part of it. You might almost think—
> Helena: What?
> Dr. Gall: That nature was offended at the manufacture of the Robots. . . . Nothing can be done. . . . All the Universities in the world are sending in long petitions to restrict the manufacture of the Robots. Otherwise, they say, mankind will become extinct through lack of fertility. But the R.U.R. shareholders, of course, won't hear of it. All the governments in the world are even clamouring for an advance in production, to raise the man-

---

* The Brothers Čapek, *R. U. R. and the Insect Play* (London: Oxford University Press, 1961), p. 9.

power of their armies. All the manufacturers in the world are ordering Robots like mad. Nothing can be done. . . .

Helena: And has nobody demanded that the manufacture should cease altogether?

Dr. Gall: God Forbid. It'd be a poor look-out for him.

Helena: Why?

Dr. Gall: Because people would stone him to death. You see, after all, it's more convenient to get your work done by Robots.

Helena: Oh, Doctor, what's going to become of people? *

The current answer to Helena's question is that people are, as in *R.U.R.,* destroying their relationship to their natural ecological environment because it is more immediately convenient to get their work done by a variety of robot machines even though this continued pattern might ultimately eliminate people. As in *R.U.R.,* people may become extinct, leaving sterile machines in their wake.

The annihilation of humanity by machines that are now *in control* is no longer in the province of the literary speculation of Čapek in *R.U.R.,* Huxley in *Brave New World,* or Orwell in *1984.* As one example, of many, the management of current doomsday machines seems to be slipping out of control:

A REPORT ON DOOMSDAY MACHINES

The world's political leaders are already losing control of their weapons—to computers—an international group of weapon scientists, including both Americans and Russians, will report today.

Their warning of an approaching day of Doctor Strangelove-style war—war in which programmed machines and not presidents or premiers pull the nuclear trigger—will be presented to an international scientists' assembly here. . . . The previously unpublicized weapons report is the summary of a . . . conference on new technology and the arms race . . . according to this summary, 26 experts on arms technology—including several from the Soviet Union—felt that:

There is already "growing dependence of [arms] systems on complex and rapid computer-controlled response and consequent erosion of the control of political leaders over final decision.

---

* Čapek, *R. U. R. and the Insect Play,* p. 15.

In the extreme, [this] could lead to systems which would be triggered on warning of attack, thereby placing the fate of the superpowers and the world entirely in the hands of radars and other sensors, and of the computers and technicians which control and interpret them.

San Francisco Chronicle
Sept. 9, 1970

The problem of the physical machine takeover of the destiny of people is obviously a phenomenon of enormous proportion. An even greater problem, one that is more subtle and insidious, exists. This involves the growing dehumanization of people to the point where they have become the walking dead. This dehumanized level of existence places people in roles in which they are actors mouthing irrelevant platitudes, experiencing programmed emotions with little or no compassion or sympathy for other people. People with this condition suffer from the existential disease of robopathology. In a society of robopaths, violence reaches monstrous proportions, wars are standard accepted practice, and conflict abounds. The problems, of course, begin with the dominant type of person in a society.

Robopaths have what Kierkegaard called "the sickness unto death." A robopath is a human who has become socially dead. Robopaths are people who function in terms of a pseudoimage. They are automatons who may appear turned-on to other people but are in fact egocentric and without true compassion. Robopaths are the reverse of Čapek's technological robots: they are people who simulate machines; their existential state is ahuman.

There are at least eight identifiable and interrelated characteristics that may help to define the more general phenomenon of the robopath, the basic pathology that psychodrama, in its form of dealing with more obvious human problems, ultimately attempts to counteract. These include: (1) ritualism, (2) past-orientation, (3) conformity, (4) image-domination, (5) acompassion, (6) hostility, and (7) alienation. These are all problem areas that require and can be controlled through psychodramatic treatment in its more universal impact.

Ritualism. Robopaths enact ritualistic behavior patterns in the context of precisely defined and accepted norms and rules. Robopaths have a limited ability to be spontaneous, to be creative, to change direction, or to modify their behavior in terms of new conditions. (This counterpoint of behavior is the primary expectation of a protagonist in psychodrama.) They are comfortable with the all-encompassing social machine definitions for behavior. Even the robopath's most emotional behavior becomes ritualistic and programmed. Sex, violence, hostility, and recreation are all preplanned, prepackaged activities, and robopaths respond on cue. The frequency, quality, and duration of most robopaths' behavior is predetermined by societal definition.

This condition perpetuates an existence in which people do not use their humanistic capacities. Their activities are rote in quality. Social interaction is a dull routine that has limited intellectual or emotional meaning.

Past-orientation. Robopaths are oriented to the past, rather than to the here-and-now situation or to the future. In this regard, they suffer from a personal form of cultural lag. They are often responding to situations and conditions that are no longer relevant or functional. They have impaired and limited vision for future emergencies. Psychodrama can unlock this rigidity by shaking a person out of his time orientation (as, for example, in the described session of the lady locked into her problem with her dead husband).

A deadly arch example of this condition of being locked into the past on a broader societal level is the continued mass individual use of the internal combustion gasoline automobile as a means of transportation. The evidence is overwhelming that the oil power needed to operate this atavistic relic is finite and disappearing, and that most people are dying slowly and some rapidly from smog; yet there is no fundamental modification of the escalation of the rigid behavior that perpetuates this no longer viable deadly machine. The robopaths in government, those in charge of the deadly automobile producing companies, and the oil companies, are more concerned with sustaining profits than with human life; and the people who buy and drive these automotive death machines are powerless to change their susceptibility to the auto industry's powerful and seductive advertising, which feeds their egos. Driving the "right," "in" car, the perpetuation of an outmoded "image" sold by mass advertising, is more important to most people than the death-machines' ecological impact or their growing lack of practicality.

In a very real sense, people's addiction to automobiles is more *deadly* than heroin addiction in the larger society. Yet because of the robopathic set to a past-orientation, we continue on our increasingly deadly path of reliance on the automobile for travel.

Conformity and Obedience to Authority. Robopaths have limited spontaneity or creativity, according to Moreno's definition of spontaneity and creativity in interaction as "a new response to an old situation and an adequate response to a new situation." Robopaths are unable to be creative in old situations or to change direction for new situations.

In a robopath-producing social machine, *conformity* is a virtue. New or different behavior is viewed as strange and bizarre. "Freaks" are feared. Originality is suspect. Consequently, the social system is seldom geared to fostering or developing a person's ability to be spontaneous and creative. Robopaths are obedient to orders from people in authority. One classic set of psychodramatic research experiments that reveals this syndrome is the work of psychologist Stanley Milgram at Yale University in the early 1960s. In his psychodramatically oriented research, Milgram studied the socially important phenomonon of robopathic obedience to authority by means of an ingenious set of role-playing situation tests.*

In his overall project, during a period of several years, almost a thousand adults were the subjects of his research. He investi-

___

* For a more comprehensive analysis of this research and its implications see Stanley Milgram, *Obedience to Authority* (New York: Harper & Row, 1974).

gated a variety of experimental settings and variable modifications. The results, however, were frighteningly uniform. On the basis of his research, Milgram concluded that a majority of "good people," who in their everyday lives were responsible and decent, could be made to perform "callous and severe" acts on other people when they were placed in situations that had the "trappings of authority." The "harsh acts" included giving electric shocks to another individual who might have just died of a heart attack. The following detailed example of one of Milgram's projects more graphically illustrates the general research approach that was used.

The subjects in this prototype example of the Milgram experiments on obedience were a random sample of New Haven adult males who came to Milgram's Yale Research Center in response to a newspaper advertisement. They were paid by the hour and individually brought to a laboratory and introduced to their partners, who were, in reality, members of the research team. Each was then told, incorrectly, that he was going to participate in a learning experiment with his partner. One of them was to be the "teacher" and the other the "learner." It was contrived that the subject always wound up as the teacher, and the research assistant always became the learner. The subject was incorrectly told that the research was being conducted to determine the effects of punishment on learning.

The subject, now the teacher, witnessed the standard procedure by which the learner (in reality, a member of the research staff) was strapped into a chair that apparently had electrical connections. The subject was then taken into another room and told to ask the learner certain questions from a questionnaire he was given. The teacher was told to administer electric shocks every time the learner gave a wrong answer. (In some cases, before the learner was strapped into his *electric* chair, he would comment, "Take it easy on me, I have a heart condition.")

In the room with the teacher was another member of the research team who served as an authority figure and as a provocateur. He was present to make sure that the subject administered the proper shocks for incorrect answers.

The subject (protagonist) was told by the authority figure to give progressively stronger shocks to the learner (auxiliary ego) when the latter's answers were incorrect. In front of the subject was an elaborate electric board that, as far as the subject knew, controlled shock levels from 15 to 450 volts in 15-volt gradations. The last two switches were ominously labeled XXX.

The researcher in the room would admonish the subject to increase the shock for each incorrect answer. In a short time, the subject was repeatedly, as far as he knew, giving shocks of up to 450 volts to another person in the next room. The "victim" would often dramatically pound the wall and shout, "Stop it, you're killing me!" Some subjects balked at continuing but proceeded on the orders of the researcher in the room, who would simply say, "Continue the experiment."

At a certain point, the "victim," after pounding on the wall, would "play dead," or act as if he had passed out, and make no sound. The researcher in the room would instruct the subject to count "no response" as an incorrect answer. He would then order him to continue to shock an apparently inert or dead body with heavy electric shocks.

In several cases, when the subject refused to act out his robopathic behavior of continuing to shock the victim because "Christ, I don't hear him anymore, maybe I killed him! You know he said he had a bad heart," the researcher would say, "Go on with the experiment." The authoritative voice of the *Yale* researcher caused more than half of the subjects to continue to robopathically shock what might very well have been a dead body!

In another part of the experiment, some subjects refused to go on. The researcher would tell the subject to continue, and say, "Go ahead, I'll be responsible for what happens to the 'learner.'" When this was done, the subject would usually say, "O.K., I'll continue. Remember you're responsible, not me!"

One of Milgram's experiments, conducted with forty subjects, is typical of those overall experiments carried out with almost one thousand people. All forty subjects complied by shocking their "victims" with up to 300 volts. Fourteen stopped at that point or at slightly higher levels. But the majority—twenty-six subjects —continued to administer increasingly more severe shocks until they reached 450 volts. This was beyond the switch marked *Danger: Severe Shock.* Thus, 65 percent of this representative sample of "good people," paid a few dollars an hour, conformed to the dictates of an experimental authority situation to the point at which *they supposedly inflicted severe pain or possible death on another human being.*

Essentially, the research validated the assumption that people would conform to the dictates of people in authority even when they knew they were inflicting severe harm on another person, up to and beyond homicide. Authority, in a legitimate social context, thus produced obedience and conformity to ahuman goals.

One of the most horrendous examples of a human "obedience to authority" in American history was the behavior of Lt. William Calley and members of his platoon at My Lai during the Vietnam War. The end point of their behavior reveals that a country that prides itself on being humanistic can produce robopathic conformists who will enact the role of cold-blooded killers.

Lt. Calley's first platoon of Charlie Company, First Battalion, Twentieth Infantry of the American Army, swept into the Vietnamese hamlet of My Lai. They left in their wake hundreds of dead civilians, including women and children. Several small children with bullet-punctured diapers were later photographed lying dead in the dust.

The perpetrators of this horrendous act, later legally defined as a war crime, were not psychotics or psychopaths but a representative sample of typical American young men, most of whom had been involuntarily drafted into the army. One of the American soldiers who participated in the killings that day later commented:

> You know when I think of somebody who would shoot up women and children, I think of a real nut, a real maniac, a

real psycho; somebody who has just completely lost control and doesn't have any idea of what he's doing. That's what I figured. That's what I thought a nut was. Then I found out [at My Lai] that an act like, you know, murder for no reason, that could be done by just about anybody.

The young men at My Lai were apparently not too different from the typical Americans in the Milgram experiments who, under orders, shocked people (from their perception) to their death. Nor were they apparently very different from the spectators who passively played their spectator role of watching people being murdered, as did the thirty-eight robopathic people who felt no obligation to intervene in the stabbing to death of Kitty Genovese in New York City.

The point is that the robopathic response, which can be an act of commission or omission, can be built into people in so-called civilized social systems. People can be, and apparently are, subtly trained to "carry out orders" or play their roles even when such orders or roles entail horrendous acts. The acts I am referring to are acts without compassion, acts that more or less kill people. These robopathic-acompassionate acts are not always deadly. There are levels of acompassionate murder that can run anywhere from unwarranted small, biting sarcasm to the ultimate act of homicide.

The rationalization or self-justification for attacks (small or large) on humanity are generally found in the context of the system. Eichmann's classic comment about "only doing his job" has been echoed by other robopathic killers. Consider the explanation of Lt. Calley in accounting for his personal and indirect killings at My Lai, including his shooting to death of a wounded baby who was attempting to crawl out of a ditch:

> I had tremendous amounts of adrenalin flowing through my body. . . . There was a strong anxiety; I think, that always goes along in situations like that. I was ordered to go in there and destroy the enemy. That was my job on that day. . . . I did not sit down and think in terms of men, women and children. They were all classified the same, and that was the classification that we dealt with—just as enemy soldiers. I felt then, and I still do,

that I acted as I was directed, and I carried out the orders that I was given, and I do not feel wrong in doing so. . . .

Lt. Calley was convicted of his crimes, even though the chain of command and guilt up to the incumbent President was legally ignored. In fact, the immediate President, Richard Nixon, saw fit to mitigate Calley's conviction by releasing him from jail until the appeal was concluded. Perhaps this was done because one robopathic personality, Nixon, could readily understand the acompassionate behavior of another, Calley, to carry out ahuman orders in the line of duty. Additionally, the silent majority of robopathic personalities around the country broke their silence and howled their disapproval of the conviction of one of their people. The robopathic majority apparently found its ideal war hero— who was later released from prison.

A national poll at the time of Calley's conviction revealed that about 75 percent of the population disagreed with the decision. The common theme expressed was that Calley was "acting under orders." The majority apparently believes that atrocities within the proper normative social framework are not deviant, and therefore are not true atrocities.

As often occurs in the case of people who are projected into the spotlight, there was a retrospective "case history" examination of Lt. Calley's growing-up process. The evidence did not reveal any spectacular traumas of an abnormal family or unusual life experiences. Calley was brought up in an average American family, went to standard schools, and lived in typical American communities. Lt. Calley was obviously not a deviant weirdo, hippie, commie, pinko, revolutionary freak. Perhaps his high school principal summed it up best when he complimented Calley's behavior in high school: "Rusty was not brilliant, but he did what he was told."

Image-Domination. Robopaths are "other-directed" rather than "inner-directed." In David Riesman's terms, they are attempting to determine what is appropriate as defined by the status definition and rules provided by those around them rather than by having any inner radar or principles to determine their behavior.

They are constantly attempting to be super-conformists. Their presentation of self is geared to others rather than to any self principles. They have limited or no interior definition for their behavioral enactments. Their behavior is thus dominated by the image requirements set up by the surrounding society.

Image-dominated people have created social rituals and artifacts that render them important in terms of their natural spontaneity and creativity. They trade their spontaneity and courage for the security of a robot role with the built-in approval of being stylish or "in."

In this regard, in hundreds of psychodrama sessions that I have directed with image-dominated people, I have concluded that many people who view themselves as "hip" or "beautiful" people are outrageous robopaths. Image-dominated people are consumed with determining the latest "in" fashions. They will acquire the "in" material objects or clothes (whether or not they can afford them) because they must maintain the fashion *image,* which provides them with immediate gratification, temporal identity, and a refuge from the necessity of confronting themselves or life's realities. Being "in" is an acceptable shield from being oneself, and if the image-dominated robopath slavishly conforms, he achieves automatic approval.

In this context, a woman TV writer once told me a story about how she acquired a contract to write a TV drama. "I received a phone call and was given an appointment for that afternoon with this important producer. I had heard from several friends what a stickler he was on status symbols and fashion. So that morning I ran all over Beverly Hills and put together a smashing outfit. You may not believe this, but when his door opened he looked me over and said melodically, 'Well, Giorgio and Gucci, come right *on* in!' He identified every new 'in' thing I bought and never mentioned my name once. Of course, I got the assignment." In a very real sense, the person did not get the writing assignment —her image did.

Another "in" personal acquaintance, in tandem with her image-dominated husband, at a party I attended made sure to inject the fact that she was into the latest everything. She injected her status symbols at the slightest pretext. In a discussion of the misbehavior of children, she let us know that "yesterday my kid got cooky crumbs all over our Oriental carpets." When the conversation veered to the manner in which children are careless, the husband commented: "Oh, it's just awful the trouble they get into. Johnny left his bike in the driveway. My dad was backing out, and his Rolls-Royce ran right over Johnny's new eight-speed French bike."

The image-dominated peoples' movement with all the fashionable name tags enables other "in" people to recognize immediately that they are O.K. Given this, there are no additional requirements—such as humanistic actions—required from the image-dominated role-players. This accounts, in part, for the unbelievably dull, flat quality of life in the places or situations where image-dominated robopaths congregate. Most of the interaction revolves around a series of acknowledgments regarding who is wearing what, going where, or acquiring a range of desirable material objects. Of greatest importance is projecting *the correct image rather than the human being.*

Image-dominated people are generally lacking in spontaneity and creativity in their verbal interaction and communication with others. Most have a frozen repertoire of conversation. When they are "running their story," it may even be charming and intelligent. The problem is that it is often the only "story" they have. After it has been delivered, or if they are pressed for elaboration, they have no spontaneity or creativity to enlarge the scope of their image-presentation. In this context, their human script is frozen into a robopathic art that may be clever on the surface but is dead at its center.

In the image-dominated syndrome, transiency is characteristic. After the "in-groupies" deliver their repertoire of wit and fashion, they must move on to other groups or persons. Their frozen act no longer produces rave notices, and they insatiably require a new set and audience.

This is especially true of the image-dominated "playboy" or

"playgirl" robopath I have directed in hundreds of psychodramas. In their love affairs, after their opening act has been presented, the next step requiring human intimacy is avoided. The avoidance emanates from an inadequacy to function at this next level, or because the person fears that his transient partner will find out there is nothing in back of the image. Psychodrama can often counterattack this problem by freeing people to become more spontaneous and compassionate.

Acompassion. If compassion entails a true concern for the human interests of others, robopaths are acompassionate. Their enactments are generally neither against other people nor for other people in terms of a sense of personal moral values or principles. They act—essentially in terms of what is most expedient behavior—to further or conform with their projected image. They will thus most often conform to the rules and the expectations of the majority. They do not have inner humanistic values that dictate or define their behavior. In psychodrama we see how they act out their role "properly" regardless of the destructive impact it may have on other people. Their role, therefore, and its "proper" enactment, becomes paramount to any concern for other people. In psychodrama, through such devices as role reversal, in which people actually take the role of another, we can sometimes modify this acompassionate characteristic. Even a person who has suffered deeply at the hands of another (e.g., the several psychodrama examples of youths oppressed by their parents) can be turned around from deep hostility to compassion by learning how to properly take the role of the other person in his life.

Hostility. Hostility, both *covert* and *overt,* is a significant characteristic of a society of robopaths and is a quality found in robopathic people. People unable to act out their spontaneity and creativity develop repressed, venomous pockets of hostility. In some robopathic roles—as, for example, soldier—there is a built-in escape valve for the aggressive build-up that would emerge from being a member of a war machine: the soldier can kill the enemy. Many bureaucrats also often have an acceptable structure for ventilating their hostility on other people. They can use the rules to deny others things they desire (e.g., "The rules do not permit . . ." "We regret we can't deliver . . ." etc.).

Robopaths can also ventilate their hostility more openly. There are innumerable cases of violent homicidal outbursts by people who have been "model citizens" or "model students" and who explode dramatically (e.g., Charles Whitman, who killed fifteen people and wounded thirty-four more from a tower at the University of Texas; Charlie Starkweather, the "good boy" who killed nine people; or Juan Corona, the nice, quiet man who murdered over twenty-five migrant farm workers, etc.).

Another apparent sign of the times is the phenomenon of Watergate. Many members of the Watergate gang acompassionately followed the orders of their arch robopathic leader. Their compliance revealed no inner radar of values but a blind conformance to the moral imbecility of their accepted leader.

Social death is akin to physical death. Robopathic people whose lives and interactions lack humanism are emotionally dead. Their responses to war, suffering, even the physical death of others are basically acompassionate, even though they may overtly appear to "care." This sophisticated and dissolute pattern of alienation seems to be another symptom of the robopathic existence.

The robopathic, acompassionate response to hostility and violence is related to Camus' *The Rebel,* in which he deals with the issue of death as a prosaic condition in which homicide and the "sanctified value of life" have become "a bore" to the masses. Camus writes:

> The poets themselves, confronted with the murder of their fellow men, proudly declare that their hands are clean. The whole world absentmindedly turns its back on these crimes; the victims have reached the extremity of their disgrace: they are a bore. In ancient times the blood of murder at least produced a religious horror and in this way sanctified the value of life. The real condemnation of the period we live in is, on the contrary, that it leads us to think that it is not bloodthirsty enough. Blood is no longer visible; it does not bespatter the faces of our pharisees

visibly enough. This is the extreme of nihilism; blind and savage murder becomes an oasis, and the imbecile criminal seems positively refreshing in comparison with our highly intelligent executioners.*

The mass robopathic response to Lt. Calley's alleged war crimes reveals, in part, the increasingly ahuman response to death. The "highly intelligent" political executioners continue their remote killing, partly because of the apathy of a mass society of robopaths.

Adolf Eichmann (a classic robopathic hero), for example, was most self-righteous about carrying out the job of "exterminating undesirables." He had no time to concern himself with any inner guilt or turmoil about his role. Efficiency was the keynote.

In a similar vein, as mentioned, Lt. Calley's alleged killing of "Oriental civilians," even after the details of the horrendous crime were made public, produced a mass affirmation of his behavior by a majority.

In a broader context, many efficient robopathic parents are self-righteous about the cold and highly defined discipline they inflict on their children. As robopathic parents administer a spanking (or worse, as demonstrated by horrendous child-battering cases), they will cite certain biblical admonitions about sin or "correct behavior." They will literally whip their children into conformist shape so that they are not embarrassed in front of the neighbors by certain immoral profanity, sexual references, or "bad behavior" that negatively affects their image. They self-righteously believe they are doing the correct thing. In effect, they build their children into robopathic people in their own image.

These patterns can be defused by providing psychodramatic opportunities to act out these usually suppressed patterns of hostility. As in the case of Ralph, when the individual through role-playing has determined the source and the size and shape of his hostility, it can often be modified into positive behavior.

Alienation. Despite the general overall appearances of "to-

---

* Albert Camus, *The Rebel* (New York: Vintage Books, 1956), p. 279.

getherness," the typical robopath is in effect alienated from *self, other people,* and the *natural environment.* He or she is alienated from *self* in the sense that his or her ego is only a function of ritualistic demands—it has no intrinsic self-definition. It is a component of a social machine.

Robopaths are alienated from *other people* because their interaction with others is usually in terms of "others" as *objects* not *human beings.* They are role-objects such as children, employees, employers, another body on a bus or train, another object in the anonymous crowd. There is limited room for compassion toward objects.

A grotesque example of this kind of alienation was the cited robopathic onlooker response to the public murder of Kitty Genovese in New York City. Thirty-eight people stood by and watched this object-victim as she was stabbed to death by an assailant and were not sufficiently impelled to respond in any way to prevent her death.

Another example of this quality of alienation is observable in the contemporary "salesman personality." Many salesmen have limited compassion and are *alienated* from their clients or customers as human beings. To such salesmen, the customers are not human but are objects to be strategically manipulated for profit. Although ethical considerations are part of the veneer of the salesman personality, in practice they will sell their *product* "by any means necessary" (e.g., a recent government report listed 369 highly advertised drug products that were either useless or hazardous. One of the most heavily "sold" products is, of course, cancerous, death-dealing tobacco). The financial profit motive dehumanizes salesmen and their clients by alienating or isolating these role-players from any humanistic interaction as people. The inter-actors become robopathic objects to each other in an ahuman interaction.

Robopaths are *alienated* from their *natural environment* because they pay more attention to the plastic intervening variables of their social machines than to the natural spectacle that surrounds them. Moreover, their ritualistic, locked-in position and behavior is a methodical destroyer of the natural ecological conditions of the earth.

These are generalized problems that appear to defy solution. Through a medium like psychodrama, however, people can be brought together impromptu to focus on these problems. The Psychodrama of Adolf Eichmann, the psychodrama of a child-abuser, personalizing homicide from the abstract news article into "the living newspaper," and a psychodrama on ecological disaster are all devices for *personalizing* problems so that people can feel them more intensively, collectively enhance their humanism, and be effectively motivated to take appropriate action.

Every historical period seems to have its dominant social-psychological pathology. Freud determined that neurosis was the central emotional disorder of his time and developed his methodology of psychoanalysis in terms of the problem he encountered. In gross terms, psychosis, sociopathology, and neurosis have been widespread and significant disorders of the post-World War II period. The twenty-first century may be characterized by an epidemic of role-bound behavior or robopathology.

This behavioral syndrome has always been in some degree a destructive side effect of technological systems. As technocracies and "technological progress" accelerate, the side effect correlative impact on people appears to be a marked increase in robopathology.

The pathology appears rampant and may in time eclipse the other identifiable behavioral disorders. Robopathic behavior and existence is less apparent, more difficult to identify, and therefore more insidious than the other maladies.

Robopaths are efficient functionaries and bureaucrats. They meld into social machines, as functional cogs, in part because, as Čapek stated, "They never think of anything new and they have no soul."

Robopaths are not deviants. They super-conform to the dictates of megamachines. In this regard, they commit subtle ahuman and dehumanizing acts as a normative part of an overall system that expects limited human compassion. In the extreme, robopaths are agents who perpetuate, validate, and commit acts of social death.

A subtle characteristic of robopathology is that, like other diseases, it is not an *all-or-none phenomenon*. There are always degrees of pathology. An infected limb may or may not affect the total physiological system of a person. Also, there are obviously degrees of intensity of infection.

In a parallel way, the infected person or social system may have a partially compartmentalized condition. An individual may have a full, happy, humanistic family situation and slave in a robopathic occupational role for the other half of his life. Or the reverse may be true: the individual's home lifestyle may be a robopathic existence and he may "labor" in his relationship with his wife and child. The wife detests her robopathic housewife existence. They mouth platitudes of "relating" and "togetherness." Their sex life is a prescribed meaningless ritual they are taught to experience, often from the latest best-selling book on the subject. In another area of his life, his job turns him on. In this role, he is spontaneous and creative, carrying out work that is compassionate and meaningful for himself and other people.

Robopathology often emerges when people *cop-out* or sell-out their humanistic drive of excitement, joy, and courage to the cultural press of social machines because of fear and often an instilled sense of inadequacy. They often trade their more spontaneous creative potentials for familiar regularized rituals. In this way, they avoid putting themselves to any test from which they might be judged or emerge as inferior.

In another dimension of the robopathic phenomenon, many creative people are often corrupted by the rewards of the society. They find a groove and freeze in it. For example, many innovators —writers, theorists, teachers, architects, artists—after an initially courageous and creatively productive life, cop-out and become robopathic in their later creative attempts. They find a successful status position, receive their rewards, and ritualistically stick to it for the rest of their lives. They no longer put themselves "in harm's way" by branching out or trying a new and different approach. Their fears and lack of courage freeze them into static, uncreative roles, where they lock into a robopathic existence even though they project an image of creativity.

We often find in psychodrama that many presumably creative people feel a numbness and dissatisfaction with their life that is traceable to their frozen positions. After a session, they often feel freed to risk a different type of creative act.

Moreno's emphasis was on developing spontaneity and creativity for confronting the tendency toward the flat, stereotyped, robot-like responses that I have described here. The psychodramatic counterattack against robopathology is not easily launched, according to Moreno in *Who Shall Survive?*:

> The control of the robot is complicated for two reasons. One reason is that the robot is man's own creation. He does not meet it face to face, like he did the beasts of the jungle, measuring his strength, intelligence and spontaneity with theirs. The robot comes from within his mind, he gave birth to it. He is confounded like every parent is towards his own child. Rational and irrational factors are mixed therefore in his relationship to robots. In the excitement of creating them he is unaware of the poison which they carry; threatening to kill his own parent. The second reason is that in using robots [cultural conserves] and zoomatons man unleashes forms of energy and perhaps touches on properties which far surpass his own little world and which belong to the larger, unexplored and perhaps uncontrollable universe.*

Part of the treatment of the robot condition, advocated by Moreno, is the use of psychodramatic methods for reversing the trend toward developing robotlike personalities *at an early age.* Moreno specifically concerned himself with the educational process for children, in which there is considerable evidence that educational systems are geared to turn out robopaths.

* Moreno, "The Social Atom and Death," p. 608.

In response to the educational machines of the time, in the late twenties, Moreno attempted to develop an innovative "Impromptu School" that used psychodrama and role-playing to counterattack the educational machine impact. In a *New York Times* article (February 18, 1929), Moreno was quoted as follows on this issue:

> Children are endowed with the gift of spontaneous expression up to the age of 5, while they are still in an unconscious creative state, unhampered by the laws and customs laid down by a long succession of preceding generations. After that they fall heir to accepted methods of expression; they become imitative, turn into automatons and in a large measure are deprived of natural outlets of volitional creation. . . .
>
> Until a certain age all children's learning is spontaneously acquired. . . . Soon, however, the adult begins to introduce into the child's world subjects unrelated to its needs. The little victim from then on is pressed by many adult sophistries into learning poems, lessons, facts, songs and so on, all of which remain like a foreign substance in an organism. The child begins to accept as superior that which is taught him and to distrust his own creative life. So very early in the life of the individual there is a tendency to mar and divert creative impulses.
>
> Here the impromptu psychodrama comes to the rescue. It offers a school of training which can be practiced in the small or large group or within the family circle itself. The impromptu method concerns itself with mental and emotional states. . . . When the impromptu instructor recognizes the pupil to be lacking in a certain state, e.g., courage, joy, etc., he places him in a specific situation in which the lacking state will be emphasized. The pupil "plays" that situation, dramatizing the state impromptu. In other words, if lacking in courage, he "plays" courage until he learns to be courageous.

It is apparent that not only children, but many adults, can benefit from "playing at courage" and developing more innovative and productive responses to life.

Beyond formal education and schools, in thousands of psychodrama sessions I have directed, I have determined that an individual's family structure and relationships provide the most fundamental group for psychodramatic action. Too often the original loving, compassionate relationship of husband and wife that originally launched the family becomes converted into a ritualized interaction between two robopaths who talk to each other's images and even make love in a set formula for physical action. The parents (and the children rapidly fall in line) never really communicate or express any spontaneous, creative, or different ways of relating. This factor, more than any other, seems to account for the escalation of various problems in contemporary society.

In this genre of robopathic family, I recall a session in which a father encountered his son about his son's rebellious behavior. The father's enactment in the psychodrama seemed to be copied from a model *Father Knows Best* television melodrama. He woodenly expressed "compassion" for his son's health but was more spontaneous and self-righteous in portraying his real concern about the potential irreparable damage to the family's image if the son were ever arrested for drugs or other misbehavior. The father's performance was marked by an almost total lack of real compassionate emotion, and the son responded in kind.

After several weeks of psychodrama sessions, the father finally broke out of his robopathic armor, got down on his knees, and poured out sixteen years of repressed tears and emotions toward his son. He told him about his beautiful feelings for him when he was born, apologized for seldom spending time with him, admitted his hostilities, and asked the son to forgive him. The son wept and embraced his father and repeated his new discovery about his father, "Dad, you can feel, Dad, you can feel. . . ."

The mother joined in on the session, and, for the first time in over sixteen years of close physical proximity, the family became emotionally intimate. Through the vehicle of psychodrama, they broke out of their robopathic role-playing in their family social machine and began to communicate in a more creative and humanistic way.

Another psychodrama I ran with a forty-year-old man named Bill depicts the robopathic problems of an image-dominated man with all the totems of success, a person who was part of the army of the walking dead. Bill was successful in business, handsome, distinctively attired, properly married—with a loving mistress on the side—urbane, intelligent, and extremely miserable.

Bill's psychodrama begins with him stepping on the stage and making his self-presentation. He believes that he has acquired all the accouterments of success defined by our society. He has professional stature, earns a sizable income, claims to love and be loved by his wife and children; however, he feels an indescribable void in his life. He cannot specify what it is, but he feels empty and unfulfilled; and he sees no prospects for positive change. Life has no meaning for him. He has recently been contemplating suicide, as he puts it, "to get out of the nothingness of my life."

Bill sets up the first scene of his session. He is in his air-conditioned Mercedes, driving home from work on the freeway. His $20,000 car is getting nowhere. He looks out at dozens of other cars, driven by men whose vapid stares signal to Bill that they too seem to be going in the same direction. It seems as if the freeway goes on forever. "Where am I rushing to, anyway? There's nothing happening at home."

In a three-hour session, he role-plays himself in his most relevant relationships: with his family, at work, with the memory and reality of his dead parents, who wanted him to succeed not as a businessman but as a doctor. As he explores his inner world by objectifying it in actuality on the stage, he begins to make a series of discoveries.

He is not as honest in his human relationships as he covertly claims or likes to think. He is role-bound and "repeats and repeats and repeats" the same behavior "day after day after day." His life is consumed with buying material objects that rapidly lose their value because the styles keep changing. "I want my wife to have the latest everything, but nothing lasts. Her closets are full of imported clothes that are practically new but useless, because they're not in style now."

He reverses roles with his wife. They are in bed. In the role of his wife, Bill says, "You've become a complete bore. You never do anything new or different. Screwing you is like being in bed with a machine."

In another scene in his session, Bill reverses roles with his six-year-old son. In the role of the son, he begins to feel what it is like to look at himself as a father, and at the world from a six-year-old viewpoint. Bill in the role of his son seems shocked when he finds himself saying, "Dad, you're always so busy. You never read to me or hug and kiss me anymore. What's wrong with me?" (At this point, Bill was put back in his own role by a role reversal and responded with love and deep emotion to his son's poignant and pertinent questions.)

Bill has lost the memory of the peak experiences of his earlier life. He begins to remember and reenacts the beauty of his early courtship and romance with his wife, the early happy years of their marriage, the excitement and joy of the birth of his son. His marriage and his work have become for him empty rituals that "no longer have any point." He finds now that his whole life is devoted to perpetuating an image of himself that others envy and admire but that he abhors.

In the psychodrama of his role-bound, *robopathic existence,* he tries radical new alternatives to his life: an emotional scene reviving his marriage; a really honest discussion with his son; a scene denouncing himself and his fellow employees. His spontaneity and creativity become somewhat revived by the session. He renews his interest in his social atom of people close to him. He literally cries about his not touching or feeling the people close to him anymore. As he enacts these psychodramatic scenes of hope, he begins to revive his humanism.

The group joins in on the session, and various people reveal their points of identification with Bill. The protagonist and the group in the psychodrama experience each other in new, different, and creative ways. They touch, hug, cry, examine, speculate—in brief, they act out a deeper, more humanistic reality. Most important, the spontaneity and creativity they have experienced carries over into their "real life." The session has revived some creative and compassionate emotional forces in the man that seem to open him up further to his family, his friends, his colleagues, and the group present at the session.

The positive impact of a good psychodrama session is immediately felt by the protagonist and the group present. The session, however, automatically has a further salutary effect on the social atom of each of the individuals present. In this way, there is a broadening ripple effect of a session from the immediate situation onto the larger society. The central point here is that the constructive effects of a session on the microcosm level (e.g., individuals and their social atom, family, work groups, impromptu consciousness-raising groups, etc.) can constructively affect the macrocosm of the large society. As people, in various types of psychodrama groups, break through their image-dominated robopathic shells, they become more compassionate and are opened up to new and more humanistic perspectives on the overall larger society. This positive fallout of humanistic emotions and perspectives will engage people more and more in attempts to constructively modify some of the robopathic, deleterious aspects of family life, the educational system, government, business organizations, and the natural environment. In brief, small group sessions at the microcosmic level can open people up to their humanism, and ultimately this process can positively affect the robopathic problems that currently exist in the large society.

Potent psychodramas in psychodrama theaters and in impromptu groups tend to automatically train people for broader psychodramatic action. In this regard, Moreno has advocated a more universal use of psychodrama, a psychodrama of the streets in which people would identify with oppressed peoples and broader issues in actual life situations.

> Psychodrama is not restricted to a psychodrama theatre. Life may provoke a simple man to turn psychodramatist. . . . This is the first psychodramatic law: Put yourself into the place of a victim of injustice and share his hurt. Reverse roles with him.

You may remember the concentration camps in Auschwitz. Millions of Jews have been thrown into gas chambers and burned alive. Men, women, children. Millions of people knew about it, Germans and non-Germans, but did nothing. But there emerged during that period of the lowest depth of inhumanity, a few men who dared to challenge this action, this mass murder. They were a number of German pastors who insisted on going with the Jewish victims into the camps to suffer with them every kind of humiliation, starvation, brutality, even going into the gas chambers to be burned alive. Against the proudest of the Nazi authorities they felt their responsibility to participate with the innocent victims in the same martyrdom. And when they were not permitted to go, they were shot and died. . . . These men died as bearers of truth. . . . The bearer of truth does what he does because of his innermost desire to establish the truth and justice and love of humanity regardless of consequences. It is a moral imperative.*

In this regard, psychodrama and other spontaneous methods developed in the context of psychodrama have a broader application and linkage toward humanizing groups in everyday life—beyond their performances in a psychodrama theater. People, through the psychodramatic methods detailed here for your own impromptu groups, are encouraged to break out of their circumscribed roles, communicate more effectively, express their deeper emotional feelings, become more compassionate, and improve their humanistic performances in life.

Psychodrama, beginning with the social atom of an individual, through the sociometry of the family, and into personalizing the meaning of epic events in the larger society can, therefore, be utilized as a vehicle for humanizing people's lives. In composite, it utilizes the best attributes of theater and daily life to reveal the essence of human experience to the participants in psychodrama groups.

Psychodrama is a theater of life in which human scenarios can be raised to a higher level of consciousness and comprehension for

* Moreno, "The Social Atom and Death," p. 610.

the purpose of enlarging humanistic communication and compassion. The desired consequences of the overall psychodramatic process is the resolution of interpersonal conflicts and the development of a more satisfying and creative human existence for all people in society.

EPILOGUE

————

The Psychodramatic Journey of J. L. Moreno

THE ORIGIN, development, and meaning of psychodrama is intrinsically part of the life history of Dr. J. L. Moreno (1889–1974), founder of psychodrama, sociometry, and the group psychotherapy movement. Moreno, in his early years, planted the roots of psychodrama in the rich philosophical and psychological soil of Vienna around the turn of the century. During that period, Moreno's goal was to develop a "theatrical cathedral" for the release of the natural human spontaneity and creativity that he believed existed naturally in everyone. As early as 1910, Moreno was preoccupied with the development of this concept of a humanistic theater of life. In that period, Moreno's Theatre of Spontaneity was a place where people in groups had the opportunity to act out their deepest dreams, frustrations, aspirations, moods of aggression, and love—in brief, the range of their human emotions. Moreno's early dreams have substantially materialized into the psychodramatic form that is practiced today around the world.

In the early period of Moreno's Theatre of Spontaneity, he had a limited concern with fostering "therapy" or "mental health." These positive consequences were noted by Moreno only as side effects of the psychodramatic process. His central "idee fixe" and motivation was spiritual: to free the spontaneously creative self in a theater of life that provided an unlimited opportunity for freedom of expression.

Moreno recalled for me once how he directed what he believed was his first psychodrama at the age of four. The event took place when he was playing with a group of children in the basement of his parents' home in Vienna. He organized the group into an impromptu play in which he took the role of God and the other children were angels. They piled chairs upward toward the ceiling and Moreno sat on the top of the structure while the children circled about it, flapping their arms like wings and singing. He found the whole production satisfactory until one of the children suggested that he fly. He tried to—no doubt well warmed up to the role—and quickly found himself on the floor with a broken arm. The incident was a long way from formal psychodrama, but it contained many of the basic elements: creativity, spontaneity, catharsis, and—based on Moreno's unfortunate experience— insight.

This event may have had a significant impact on Moreno, since many years later he summed up his work for me in the following way: "My work is the psychotherapy of fallen gods. We are all fallen gods. As infants we have a godlike sense of power, what I call normal megalomania. Because everybody around the infant responds to his needs, he feels at one with the whole world. Every event seems the result of his own spontaneous creation. But as society makes its demands, our once boundless horizons shrink, we feel diminished, and our frustrations sometimes produce emotional disorders. Psychodrama helps people recover something of their primary selves, their lost godhead."

Although he had experimented with role-playing since he was a child and ran sessions with children in the gardens of Vienna when he was a teenager, formal psychodrama according to Moreno had its origins in a spontaneous theater group that he formed when he was a young man in his early twenties. There were many illustrious actors in Moreno's Vienna repertory group, including Elizabeth Bergner and Peter Lorre. One actor in the group told Moreno one day about the problems he was having with his wife. In her theatrical performances she was kind and compassionate, but her husband told Moreno that in their personal life she had a fiery temper that was destroying their relationship. Moreno, with the theatrical group present, put their marriage on stage in a session that was an embryonic psychodrama. He had the couple improvise key scenes in their life as if they were in their own home. Members of the repertory group helped the couple portray their conflict by joining in various roles. Moreno concluded from the group's intense response that the couple's enactment of their real conflict was more electrifying and productive to the group than any theatrical scene they had ever performed. Based on this experience, he began to more formally experiment with group enactments. This led to the development of people reversing roles with each other, doubling, and other methods that have become part of the psychodramatic approach since its origins.

Concurrent with his theatrical involvement, Moreno, during this period, was a formal student. He studied philosophy and medicine at the University of Vienna and in 1917 received his M.D. from the university. In those early years as a student, his philosophical heroes were Hegel, Spinoza, Jesus, and Socrates. Although he had many excellent professors at the university and was a devoted student, Moreno had a unique perspective on his education: "I had two teachers, Jesus and Socrates; Jesus the improvising saint, and Socrates, in a curious sort of way, the closest to being a pioneer of the psychodramatic format. His dialogues impressed me, not because of their content, but because they were presented as 'reports' of actual sessions."

Despite the fact that Moreno was a dedicated formal scholar in the European tradition, he always reveled in direct contact and "doubled" for people in all walks of life. He never restricted himself to an all-enveloping ivory tower existence. Among his many psychodramatic activities during this period was a unique project that he initiated with prostitutes in the brothels of Vienna. The project began when he noted how the police and the public stigmatized and mistreated prostitutes. Based on his empathy for their plight, he began to organize hundreds of them in small informal encounter groups in which they discussed their mutual problems.

In an ironic way, Moreno's learning experience from this project facilitated his formulation of some of the basic concepts of group psychotherapy. From the outside it looked like a prostitutes' "union." However, because Moreno began to see that "one individual could become a therapeutic agent of the other," the potentiality of group psychotherapy crystallized in his mind. From his experience with the community of prostitutes, he delineated three aspects of group psychotherapy that, from his viewpoint, "later became the cornerstone of all forms of group psychotherapy": (1) the necessary autonomy of the group; (2) the fact that all groups have a structure, and that group diagnosis is a prerequisite to group psychotherapy; and (3) the problem of anonymity. With regard to his latter point, Moreno asserted that "when a client is treated within the framework of individual therapy, he is alone with the doctor, his ego is the only focus, he has a name, his psyche is highly valued private property. But in group psychotherapy there is a tendency towards anonymity of membership, the boundaries between the egos weaken, the group as a whole becomes the important thing."

Moreno's concepts of psychodrama and group psychotherapy emanated from actual groups and unique personal experiences and encounters, but he wisely sharpened his social science theories over the next decade through many lengthy intellectual encounters and dialogues with the brilliant intellectual minds of

Vienna. Alfred Adler, August Aichorne, and Theodore Reich attended some of Moreno's sessions in his theatre of Spontaneity. On several occasions at the university, he met Freud and participated with him in discussions of the differences and similarities between psychoanalysis and psychodrama. Moreno rejected what he felt was the static and individualistic quality of Freud's system. He felt he could never restrict therapeutic practice to a one-to-one relationship in an office setting. He always perceived his theories as action methods; and creativity to Moreno involved "being an *actor*—rather than an *analyst*."

Moreno came to the United States in 1925 to promote an invention he was then working on, a machine for the recording and playback of sound on steel discs, which he patented in 1924 and brought with him to the United States. His interest in this form of technology later led to the earliest experiments with the recording and playback of therapist-patient sessions.

Although he was never disdainful of formal social science, he always maintained his sense of humor about scientific pomposity. When he arrived in New York, he reported that "when I was asked by a newspaper reporter what I though of American social science I replied: 'The only American social scientist I know anything about is Walt Whitman.' "

He decided to remain in the United States, was licensed, began medical-psychiatric practice in New York, and eventually became a naturalized American citizen. Immediately, he set out to introduce psychodrama into the mental health professions and into American culture in general. He began psychodramatic work with children at the Plymouth Institute in Brooklyn and also became involved with the Mental Hygiene Clinic at Mt. Sinai Hospital. In 1929 he began the first regular program of large-scale "open" psychodrama in America three times a week in an Impromptu Group Theatre at Carnegie Hall.

During this period, there was also considerable progress in sociometric research into group structure. Moreno made sociometric studies of the inmate social structure at Sing Sing Prison in

1931 and 1932; and from 1932 to 1938 he was engaged in a long-term delinquent project at the New York State Training School for Delinquent Girls at Hudson, New York.

Moreno rapidly became well known in America, both to the general public as a result of newspaper reports on his Impromptu Theatre, Living Newspaper demonstrations, and also within the psychiatric community. Much of his publicity in the latter category had to do with controversies—such as his celebrated exchange with Dr. A. A. Brill, a disciple of Freud—over what Brill claimed were "the neurotic characteristics of Abraham Lincoln." As a discussant of Brill's paper, Moreno defended the former president against Brill's long-distance psychoanalytic assault during a meeting of the American Psychiatric Association in 1931. Over the years, Moreno became a Fellow and honored member of the American Psychiatric Association.

In addition to his work at Beacon and his private practice, Moreno's writings encompassed the broad range of the social sciences. In 1948 he became a close friend personally and professionally of professor Wellman J. Warner, then head of the Sociology Department at New York University. Moreno was offered and accepted a professorship in sociology at N.Y.U. As a consequence of these circumstances, I first met Dr. Moreno in 1949 when I became a graduate student in sociology at New York University and enrolled in his seminar on psychodrama.

Moreno's course and my participation in several psychodrama sessions triggered my deeper involvement in the movement. We both had an immediate positive attraction at our first meeting, and I joined the psychodrama movement with a great enthusiasm that has remained constant all of these years. At my first private meeting with Moreno, I was offered and happily accepted a scholarship to train with him at his New York Institute and at his center in Beacon, fifty miles north of New York City.

The thing I remember most about Moreno at our early meetings in the fifties were his eyes. I never met anyone who looked at me so directly, honestly, and with such intensity. When I later read

Moreno's "Concept of the Encounter," I discovered he had written what I experienced in his presence:

> A meeting of two: eye to eye, face to face.
> And when you are near I will tear your eyes out
>   and place them instead of mine,
>   and you will tear my eyes out
>   and will place them instead of yours,
>   then I will look at you with your eyes
>   and you will look at me with mine.

From the outset, I immediately had a very direct and personal relationship with a man I felt had psychic powers and qualities. As a scientist, I have only a marginal belief in mysticism, but with Moreno I had the feeling that he had developed a form of E.S.P. I have since concluded that his perceptions and insights were not exclusively extrasensory. In part, they were based on a close understanding of the culture, human motivation, and body positions that had been revealed to him in decades of participating in psychodrama sessions.

Part of my training involved going to Beacon and helping to direct weekend workshops. In recent years, there has been "the discovery of marathons" and other weekend-type encounters. In the early fifties at Beacon, we pioneered such intensive nonstop weekend marathon workshops.

Around 1951–1952, Moreno was revising his now classic book *Who Shall Survive?*, originally published in 1934. It was my pleasure and honor to be invited by him to assist with editing the new edition, which was published in 1953. The experience was, for me, more profound than many of my formal classes in sociology and psychology at N.Y.U.—and no doubt Moreno's excitement, perception, dialogue, and spontaneous method of writing inspired me to become a writer.

A dominant theme of Moreno's was that he was a holy man, in the sense that he was whole or holistic. All of his work and all of his personal and familial relationships were part of his system. In Beacon and at N.Y.U. in those days, he had students and patients, he was writing, he was lecturing, he was learning. I had the rare opportunity to observe a blood-and-guts intellectual in action.

Moreno played his many roles with ease and charm. To me he was a highly significant intellectual role-model, and I availed myself of the opportunity to study and work with him in his varied roles. He would at one time be lecturing to a group of psychiatrists or students or working with patients in his sanitorium at Beacon or writing his books, and all of these activities were integrated with a religious zeal. Although of Jewish parentage, Moreno practiced no formal religion; yet all of his theories had religious characteristics and implications. He attempted to broaden his concept of psychiatry beyond its medical and sociological limitations and to enlarge the concept of religion beyond its historical, cultural, and theological limitations. He believed that a therapist must entwine his personal life with his theories and methods: "Therapeutic theories and methods without the physician who embodies them, able to grasp and to practice them, are meaningless and dead. And a healer without adequate theories and methods is like a painter without arms."

Another characteristic of my psychodramatic origins with Moreno was his realistic assessment of the social science view of him. Of course, he had many supportive colleagues and co-workers, but many therapists and social scientists in the 1950s were very threatened by, and hostile toward, Moreno. One has to remember that therapy in those days was still clearly an individually oriented approach. Here was Moreno talking of the importance of the group in producing personality modification and social change. He had already introduced sociometry, psychodrama, and sociodrama, and these ideas were beginning to stir up the minds and guts of all stripes of psychiatrists and psychologists.

Some of them felt threatened because much of their professional lives centered around the training and practice of an individually oriented psychotherapy. Those who saw the validity of Moreno's social science system and the necessity of having to change their direction so dramatically were often consciously and unconsciously disturbed by this prospect.

One fall evening in 1952, Moreno invited me to accompany him to a lecture on psychodrama and the group method that he was invited to give to a group of New York psychotherapists. The session took place before a group of around one hundred psycho-analysts and psychiatrist of various schools. I have never forgotten the hatred and chastisement that Moreno encountered that afternoon in response to his belief in the primacy of *group* concepts in all types of therapy. He was openly denounced, ridiculed, and even laughed at by members of the group during a brutal question and comment period at the end of his presentation. Some of the illustrious therapists loudly whispered as we left, "What a nut!" "He [Moreno] is a paranoid schiz." Moreno maintained his cool. As we traveled downtown, I said, "How can you take these insults?" He smiled, "First, Lew, I know I'm right. Secondly, I may be crazy like they say, but I'm making a lot of other people, like you, crazy with me; and each year, as more and more people join our movement, I will be considered less crazy."

In recent years, many former dissenters have jumped onto the group therapy and psychodrama bandwagon. There are still many individually oriented therapists and classical psychoanalysts; however, many of these therapists have come to recognize the validity and significance of the group process and psychodrama and the use of these concepts and methods as adjuncts to their practice.

It has been a gratifying aspect of my life to witness Moreno's impact, and, in a modest way, through my own involvement, to help change the orientation of so many people, in the brief span of some twenty-five years, to an acceptance of the validity of the group and psychodramatic viewpoint of therapy and society.

The last time I saw J. L. Moreno was shortly before he died, when I traveled to his home and training center in Beacon, New York, to say goodbye. His death was a fitting departure for the man who invented psychodrama; for Moreno, in a sense, directed his own rites.

By the end of April 1974, a series of minor strokes had weakened him. At the age of 85, he was confined to his bed, unable to walk around, and slowed down considerably in his speech. Such immobility was particularly distasteful to a man of Moreno's energy who felt that his internal basic life force and vigorous spirit were still intact. Because eating solid food was painful, and he knew he would die soon anyway Moreno decided to hasten the end and die with dignity. It was his decision to stop eating altogether, and he chose to subsist on water.

At that time, the American Society of Group Psychotherapy and Psychodrama, which Moreno had founded, was meeting in New York City. Over 2,000 professionals from all over the globe had traveled to attend the conference, and many of them had come explicitly to say goodbye to Moreno. At first, he consented to see only a few close friends. But finally he told his beloved colleague and wife, Zerka, "Let's not be negative. Say yes to everyone who wants to come to Beacon to see me."

So Moreno spent his last days propped up in bed, while hundreds of former students, friends, and professional associates filed through his bedroom one by one. Each visitor would pay his or her final respects, exchange expressions of love, and lean over to be hugged by Moreno. Moreno would then raise his fist in a power salute—a gesture that he initiated years before the black-power movement took hold—as if to tell them to carry on the good work, that it was someone else's turn.

My own feelings were mixed as I arrived in Beacon that spring afternoon. I had felt a deep sorrow the week before when Zerka called me in California to tell me that her husband might soon die. Moreno had been able to talk briefly on the phone. We joked a bit, and I entreated him to stick around until I could come to Beacon to say goodbye in person. He said matter-of-factly, "Lew, I'm ready to die, but I look forward to seeing you."

It was hard to conceive of the loss of my former teacher, second father, and friend of over twenty-five years. But when Zerka told me about J. L.'s acceptance and even encouragement of his own death, I felt a great deal of comfort. "After all," said Zerka, "he has lived a full and significant life."

When I arrived, life at Beacon was going on as usual. The peaceful New England atmosphere at Moreno's wooded country estate belied the activity in the buildings that served as a powerhouse for psychodrama training and publications. Some twenty students, who lived in a dormitory residence, were training as psychodrama directors. In another building, an office of secretaries worked on correspondence and publications of Beacon House, Inc., which has published almost all of Moreno's writings, as well as various journals of group psychotherapy and psychodrama founded by him.

When I walked into Moreno's bedroom, he had a smile of welcome on his face. We embraced and kissed, and I could feel a sob rising in my chest. "This is no time for sadness, Lew," Moreno whispered in my ear. "I've lived a full life. I've done my job. It's time for me to go on to something else."

Although he was prone, he was still my director and I was the protagonist. According to his plan—one that I more than welcomed—I spent the afternoon in the dining room, right off his bedroom, reading his as yet unpublished autobiography. Most of the episodes in Moreno's autobiography were not new to me. I was familiar with my friend's life history, since, over the years, he had told me many stories—over dinner or on the train when we traveled between New York and his Beacon sanatorium. We had long talks during summer vacation, when I sometimes stayed at the Beacon Center directing workshops and sometimes assisting him with revisions of his articles and books. Still, reading this panorama of events and insights was an overwhelming experience for me, especially when the hero of the odyssey was ten steps away. I read for five hours, stopping only to laugh with him over some humorous episode or probe a point with him.

As I approached the end of reading the autobiography, I

noted a vignette related to Freud that we both especially enjoyed. In Moreno's creative megalomania, he wrote how he had died and, of course, had gone to heaven. As part of Moreno's heavenly reward, along with other philosophers, he was allowed to participate in an eternal dialogue with some of the brilliant minds of history. On this particular day, Moreno was the subject of an intellectual trial that involved a grand rap session between Spinoza, Einstein, Hegel, Christ, Freud, and several other luminaries. The subject, of course, was the relative merits of psychodrama versus psychoanalysis. After several hours of brilliant debate, the group had reached a stalemate. One "celestial" member, noting that Freud had been strangely silent in defending his position, asked him what he thought of Moreno's psychodrama. A silence fell on the group, as they anticipated a powerful and eloquent diatribe that would elevate the merits of psychoanalysis far above those of psychodrama. Finally, Freud acknowledged stoically, "If I had lived longer, I too would have most certainly become a psychodramatist like Moreno."

Moreno and I laughed over his vision of paradise as I sat by his bedside for the last time. It was early evening, and I was preparing for my ride back to New York City with some students then in residence at Beacon. Even now, I see that final farewell as less of a definite separation and more of an evolutionary step in my relationship with Moreno. We embraced, and I left the room feeling that he was still with me.

When I direct a psychodrama or write about the method, I think about Moreno. And when I realize the freedom that psychodrama has given me and so many others, the ability to play many roles in life with a wide range of emotions and a broader intellectual perspective, I feel a closeness, not a separation, from the wonderful man who founded the movement.

INDEX

———